Medical Biller

-

The Comprehensive Guide

By

VIRUTI SHIVAN

Masters in Clinical Psychology (Major)

"In books, as in life, it's not the size or looks but

the content that matters."

Introduction

Welcome to the world of medical billing, a crucial yet often overlooked facet of the healthcare industry. This guide, **"Medical Biller - The Comprehensive Guide,"** is meticulously crafted to serve as your beacon through the intricate maze of healthcare billing and coding. Whether you're a curious newcomer eager to embark on a rewarding career or a seasoned professional aiming to polish your skills, this book is designed to cater to your every need.

Embarking on a journey into medical billing is akin to learning a new language. It's a world filled with complex terminologies, intricate procedures, and nuanced policies that can seem daunting at first glance. Yet, fear not! Our goal is to transform this journey into an engaging adventure, filled with enlightening insights and practical knowledge that you can apply in real-world scenarios.

Medical billing is the invisible engine that powers the healthcare system, ensuring that services provided by doctors, nurses, therapists, and other healthcare professionals are accurately charged and reimbursed. Behind every medical procedure lies a meticulous process of coding and billing that requires precision, attention to detail, and a deep understanding of medical and insurance regulations.

But why is medical billing so important? Imagine a world without it. Healthcare providers would struggle to get reimbursed for their services, resources would be misallocated, and patients could face incorrect charges, leading to a chaotic healthcare environment. Medical billing not only ensures the financial stability of healthcare providers but also protects patients from billing errors and insurance discrepancies.

This book is divided into chapters that cover every aspect of medical billing, from the basics of medical terminology to the complexities of dealing with insurance companies and legal compliance. Each chapter is packed with practical examples, making the learning process both informative and enjoyable. You'll find real-life scenarios that illustrate common challenges and effective strategies to overcome them. Plus, exercises at the end of each chapter will help reinforce your learning and test your understanding.

A human touch in medical billing? Absolutely! Behind every code, every invoice, and every claim, there's a patient with a story. In this guide, we'll remind you of the human aspect of medical billing – the empathy, the ethics, and the responsibility to ensure that every patient's journey through the healthcare system is as smooth and stress-free as possible.

Our journey together will be one of discovery, learning, and growth. The field of medical billing is ever-evolving, with new technologies, regulations, and practices emerging constantly. Staying informed and adaptable is key to success, and this guide aims to equip you with the knowledge and skills necessary to navigate the changes with confidence.

So, grab your highlighter, roll up your sleeves, and let's dive into the fascinating world of medical billing. Together, we'll unravel the complexities, celebrate the victories, and perhaps even have a bit of fun along the way. Welcome aboard!

Chapter 1: Understanding the Basics of Medical Billing

1.1 The Role of a Medical Biller

Welcome to the first stop on our journey through the captivating world of medical billing! Before we dive into the intricacies of codes and claims, let's start with the foundation of it all: understanding the vital role of a medical biller. This role is much more than just sending out bills and processing payments. It's about being the linchpin that connects healthcare providers, patients, and insurance companies.

What Does a Medical Biller Do?

Imagine a bustling bridge connecting three islands – one represents healthcare providers, another patients, and the third insurance companies. The medical biller is the architect, caretaker, and traffic controller of this bridge, ensuring smooth and efficient communication between all parties. Their primary responsibilities include:

- **Preparing and Submitting Claims:** Medical billers transform healthcare services into billing claims, adhering to complex coding protocols to ensure accuracy and compliance with federal and insurance regulations.

- **Verifying Patient Insurance:** They verify patients' insurance coverage, understand policy benefits, and communicate with patients about their billing responsibilities.

- **Following Up on Claims:** After submitting claims, billers track their progress, following up on denied or unpaid claims and working to resolve discrepancies.

- **Processing Payments and Adjustments:** They post payments received from insurance companies and patients, applying adjustments and refunds as necessary.

- **Customer Service:** Medical billers often serve as a critical point of contact for patients, explaining charges, insurance benefits, and payment options.

The Importance of Accuracy and Ethics

Accuracy is the heart and soul of medical billing. A single misplaced code can lead to claim denials, delayed payments, and unnecessary stress for patients and providers alike. Moreover, medical billers must navigate the fine line between maximizing reimbursements and adhering to ethical billing practices. They must be vigilant against fraud and abuse, ensuring that every claim accurately reflects the services provided.

A Day in the Life of a Medical Biller

Let's take a moment to walk in the shoes of a medical biller. Your day might start with reviewing notes from the previous day's healthcare services, updating patient records, and preparing claims for submission. Throughout the day, you'll answer calls from patients, clarifying their bills, and discussing payment options. You'll also interact with insurance companies, advocating on behalf of the healthcare provider or the patient to resolve claim issues. It's a role that demands attention to detail, problem-solving skills, and a deep understanding of medical billing codes and regulations.

Why Medical Billing?

Pursuing a career in medical billing offers a unique blend of challenges and rewards. It's a profession that provides stability, opportunities for advancement, and the satisfaction of playing a crucial role in the healthcare system. Every day, you'll be solving puzzles, translating complex medical services into the universal language of codes and claims, and ultimately, helping patients navigate the financial aspects of their healthcare journey.

As we move forward in this guide, remember that the role of a medical biller is not just about processing transactions. It's about facilitating access to healthcare, ensuring the sustainability of healthcare providers, and safeguarding the integrity of the billing process. Your work as a medical biller has a profound impact on the well-being of patients and the efficiency of our healthcare system.

1.2 Introduction to Medical Terminology

As we venture further into the realm of medical billing, we encounter the backbone of the healthcare industry: medical terminology. This language, rich and precise, allows healthcare professionals to communicate with unmatched clarity and efficiency. For medical billers, understanding this language is not just beneficial; it's essential. It's the key to unlocking accurate billing, ensuring compliance, and fostering effective communication.

The Alphabet Soup of Healthcare

Medical terminology can feel like an alphabet soup, with acronyms and abbreviations swirling around. From diagnoses (ICD codes) to procedures (CPT and HCPCS codes), each term, abbreviation, and code carries significant meaning. These terms are derived from Latin and Greek, providing a universal language that transcends regional dialects and languages. Here's why diving into this "soup" is crucial for medical billers:

- **Accuracy in Coding:** Knowing the difference between similar-sounding terms (e.g., "hypertension" vs. "hypotension") ensures that the right codes are applied, which is crucial for accurate billing and avoiding claim denials.

- **Effective Communication:** Understanding medical terminology allows billers to communicate effectively with healthcare providers, insurance companies, and patients, bridging any gaps in understanding.

- **Compliance and Advocacy:** Familiarity with medical terms helps billers ensure compliance with healthcare laws and advocate for providers and patients in disputes over coverage and reimbursement.

Breaking Down Medical Terms

Medical terminology is structured in a way that makes it easier to understand once you grasp the basics. Most terms consist of a root word (the base of the term), prefixes (added to the beginning), and suffixes (added to the end). For example, in the term "neurology" ('neuro-' meaning nerve and '-logy' meaning study of), we're talking about the study of the nervous system.

- **Root Words** tell the main story of the term, indicating the part of the body or the system involved.

- **Prefixes** can denote location, time, number, or status, adding important details to the root word.

- **Suffixes** often describe a condition, disease process, or procedure, completing the picture.

A Practical Approach to Learning Medical Terminology

Embarking on the journey to master medical terminology might seem daunting, but it's more like learning a new language one step at a time. Here are a few strategies:

- **Start with the Basics:** Focus on common prefixes, suffixes, and root words. This foundation will help you decode many medical terms.

- **Use Flashcards:** A tried-and-true method for memorizing terms. Regular review can dramatically improve your retention.

- **Apply What You Learn:** Practice by coding real medical scenarios or by taking exercises designed to reinforce your understanding.

- **Stay Curious:** Whenever you encounter a new term, take a moment to break it down. This active engagement with the material enhances learning.

The Human Touch in Medical Terminology

While medical terminology is scientific and precise, it serves a deeply human purpose: to ensure that every patient receives accurate and effective care. For medical billers, each term coded is more than just a string of letters; it represents a person, a treatment, and a step towards healing. Your commitment to understanding this language reflects your role in the compassionate delivery of healthcare.

In conclusion, medical terminology is not just a tool of the trade for medical billers—it's a bridge to greater understanding, efficiency, and empathy within the healthcare system. As we continue our journey through the comprehensive guide to medical billing, let this introduction to medical terminology serve as your first step towards mastering the art and science of this essential field.

1.3 Overview of Healthcare Systems

Venturing deeper into the intricacies of medical billing requires a broad understanding of the environment in which it operates: the healthcare system. This vast network, composed of hospitals, clinics, insurance companies, government agencies, and other healthcare providers, is as complex as it is crucial to society's well-being. An overview of this system not only lays the groundwork for proficient medical billing but also illuminates the interconnectedness of various stakeholders in the delivery of healthcare.

The Structure of Healthcare Systems

At its core, the healthcare system is designed to meet the health needs of individuals and populations. However, the structure and functionality of these systems can vary significantly from country to country and even within regions. Broadly speaking, healthcare systems can be categorized into several types:

- **Single-Payer Systems:** In these systems, a single public or quasi-public agency organizes health care financing, but the delivery of care remains largely in private hands. Examples include Canada and the United Kingdom.

- **Multi-Payer Systems with Universal Coverage:** These systems, found in countries like Germany and Japan, feature multiple insurance providers but offer universal coverage, often regulated by the government to ensure comprehensive access.

- **Private Insurance Systems:** In some countries, such as the United States, healthcare is primarily financed through private insurance, with government programs covering specific groups like the elderly and low-income populations.

- **Out-of-Pocket Models:** In many parts of the world, particularly in less developed countries, healthcare services are paid for directly by the patients, leading to significant barriers to access.

The Role of Insurance in Healthcare

Insurance plays a pivotal role in healthcare systems, acting as a mediator between healthcare providers and patients. It serves multiple functions:

- **Risk Pooling:** Insurance spreads the financial risk of health expenses across many individuals, making healthcare costs more predictable and manageable.

- **Access Facilitation:** By covering a portion or the entirety of healthcare costs, insurance facilitates access to necessary medical services.

- **Quality and Efficiency:** Insurance companies often advocate for quality and efficiency in healthcare delivery, negotiating prices and setting standards for care.

Healthcare Providers and Facilities

Healthcare systems are comprised of a variety of providers and facilities, each playing a unique role in delivering care:

- **Primary Care:** Often the first point of contact, primary care providers offer comprehensive health services, including prevention, diagnosis, and treatment of common illnesses.

- **Specialty Care:** Specialist providers offer services in specific areas of medicine, such as cardiology or neurology, typically requiring a referral from a primary care provider.

- **Hospitals and Clinics:** These facilities provide a broad range of services, from emergency care to surgery and rehabilitation.

- **Long-Term Care Facilities:** Nursing homes and assisted living facilities offer long-term care services for individuals who require ongoing assistance with daily activities.

Challenges and Opportunities

Healthcare systems worldwide face a myriad of challenges, including rising costs, unequal access to services, and the need for innovation in care delivery. However, these challenges also present opportunities for improvement and reform. Medical billers, positioned at the intersection of healthcare delivery and financing, play a crucial role in navigating these challenges, advocating for fair and accurate billing practices, and ensuring the sustainability of healthcare providers.

The Human Element

At its heart, the healthcare system is about people—caring for them, healing them, and improving their quality of life. For medical billers, understanding the complexities of the healthcare system is not just about mastering procedures and codes; it's about contributing to a system that upholds the dignity, respect, and health of every individual. As we continue to explore the facets of medical billing, remember that each claim processed and each code entered is a part of a larger effort to deliver compassionate and effective care.

1.4 Exercise: 10 MCQs with Answers at the End

Test your knowledge of the fundamentals of medical billing with these multiple-choice questions (MCQs). These questions are designed to reinforce your understanding of the topics covered in Chapter 1, including the role of a medical biller, medical terminology, the overview of healthcare systems, and more.

Questions:

1. What is the primary role of a medical biller?

   A) Diagnosing patient illnesses

   B) Prescribing medications

   C) Preparing and submitting healthcare claims

   D) Providing direct patient care

2. Which of the following is a key component of medical terminology?

   A) Internet slang

   B) Medical abbreviations

   C) Musical notations

   D) Culinary terms

3. In a single-payer healthcare system, who is responsible for healthcare financing?

   A) Multiple private insurance companies

   B) Patients, through out-of-pocket payments

   C) A single public or quasi-public agency

   D) Non-governmental organizations

4. Which term describes the systematic study of the structure and diseases of the nervous system?

A) Cardiology

B) Oncology

C) Neurology

D) Gastroenterology

5. What is the primary purpose of insurance in healthcare?

A) To provide employment for healthcare workers

B) To design new medical equipment

C) To spread financial risk among many individuals

D) To build more hospitals

6. Which of the following best describes a multi-payer system with universal coverage?

A) Healthcare is financed by a single government-run program.

B) Private companies offer insurance plans regulated by the government.

C) All medical services are paid directly by the patients.

D) Healthcare providers are exclusively private entities.

7. What does a medical biller use to transform healthcare services into billing claims?

A) A calculator

B) Medical billing codes

C) A stethoscope

D) Personal judgment and intuition

8. The process of verifying patient insurance coverage is essential for:

A) Determining eligibility for medical services

B) Calculating the hospital's yearly budget

C) Designing new medical procedures

D) Recruiting new healthcare professionals

9. HIPAA compliance is important for medical billers to ensure:

A) Patient entertainment

B) The speed of service delivery

C) Patient privacy and data security

D) The color scheme of medical documents

10. Which of the following is a challenge faced by healthcare systems worldwide?

A) Decreasing healthcare demands

B) Lowering technology costs

C) Rising healthcare costs

D) Excessive healthcare facilities

Answers:

1. C) Preparing and submitting healthcare claims

2. B) Medical abbreviations

3. C) A single public or quasi-public agency

4. C) Neurology

5. C) To spread financial risk among many individuals

6. B) Private companies offer insurance plans regulated by the government.

7. B) Medical billing codes

8. A) Determining eligibility for medical services

9. C) Patient privacy and data security

10. C) Rising healthcare costs

Chapter 2: Navigating Health Insurance

2.1 Types of Health Insurance Plans

As we embark on the second chapter of our journey through the world of medical billing, we delve into the labyrinth of health insurance. Understanding the types of health insurance plans is crucial for medical billers, as it influences every aspect of billing, from the coding of services to the processing of claims. Health insurance plans come in various shapes and sizes, each with its own set of rules, benefits, and limitations. Let's navigate through the most common types of health insurance plans, shedding light on their characteristics and how they impact the billing process.

Health Maintenance Organization (HMO) Plans

Imagine a tightly knit community where everyone knows each other, and there's a strong sense of structure. That's the essence of an HMO plan. Members of an HMO plan must choose a primary care physician (PCP) who acts as the gatekeeper to specialist services and hospital care. The catch? Care must be received from providers within the HMO's network to be covered, fostering a focus on preventive care and coordination.

Preferred Provider Organization (PPO) Plans

PPO plans offer a bit more freedom compared to HMOs, akin to having a VIP pass that lets you skip the line. With a PPO, you can see any doctor or specialist without needing a referral, including those outside the plan's network, though at a higher cost. This flexibility makes PPO plans a popular choice for those who value choice and convenience in their healthcare.

Exclusive Provider Organization (EPO) Plans

EPO plans strike a balance between HMO and PPO plans. Like PPOs, they allow members to see specialists without a referral. However, like HMOs, care must be received from within the plan's network (except in emergencies), blending network savings with direct access to specialists.

Point of Service (POS) Plans

POS plans are the chameleons of health insurance, offering features of both HMO and PPO plans. You're required to choose a primary care physician who will coordinate your care and provide referrals to in-network specialists. Yet, you also have the option to seek care outside the network at a higher out-of-pocket cost, providing a flexible, albeit more complex, approach to healthcare access.

High Deductible Health Plan (HDHP) with Health Savings Account (HSA)

HDHPs are the minimalist's approach to health insurance, characterized by higher deductibles but lower monthly premiums. Paired with a Health Savings Account (HSA), they allow you to save money, tax-free, to be used for medical expenses. This plan encourages consumers to make more informed health care decisions, offering significant savings for those who are healthy and have fewer medical needs.

Understanding the Impact on Medical Billing

Each type of health insurance plan has its own billing intricacies. For instance, billing an HMO might require additional documentation to prove that the provided services were necessary and within the network. On the other hand, PPO billing might involve negotiating reimbursements for out-of-network services. EPO and POS plans add layers of complexity with their unique rules for network and referral requirements. Lastly, billing for HDHPs often involves coordinating with HSAs, requiring a deep understanding of deductible management and patient payment responsibilities.

For medical billers, mastering the details of these plans is not just about ensuring accurate billing; it's about navigating a vital aspect of patient care. By understanding the nuances of each health insurance plan, medical billers can better advocate for patients, ensuring they receive the care they need within the confines of their insurance coverage. This knowledge also empowers billers to anticipate potential billing issues, streamline the claims process, and contribute to a more efficient and patient-centered healthcare experience.

2.2 Insurance Terms and Policies

Diving deeper into the realm of health insurance, we encounter a tapestry of terms and policies that form the fabric of the industry. For medical billers and anyone navigating the healthcare system, understanding these terms is akin to holding a map in a complex maze. It empowers you to make informed decisions, communicate effectively with insurance providers, and ensure accurate billing practices. Let's unravel some of the essential insurance terms and policies you'll encounter on this journey.

Premium

Think of the premium as the entry fee to the world of health insurance. It's the amount you pay, typically on a monthly basis, to keep your insurance policy active. Whether you use medical services or not, this fee ensures that you're covered when you need it.

Deductible

The deductible is your financial co-pilot on the road to insurance coverage. It's the amount you need to pay out of pocket for your medical services before your insurance plan starts to pay its share. High deductible plans often have lower premiums, appealing to those who prefer lower monthly costs in exchange for a higher upfront payment on services.

Co-payment (Co-pay)

Co-pay is the small fee that acts as your ticket each time you visit a doctor, specialist, or require a prescription drug. It's a fixed amount and varies depending on the type of service or medication. Co-pays are a way of sharing the cost of your care and are typically due at the time of service.

Co-insurance

After you've met your deductible, co-insurance is the percentage of the cost of your medical care that you share with your insurance company. For example, if your co-insurance is 20%, you pay 20% of the cost of a medical visit, and your insurance covers the remaining 80%. This cost-sharing mechanism continues until you reach your out-of-pocket maximum.

Out-of-Pocket Maximum

This term is your financial safety net. The out-of-pocket maximum is the most you'll have to spend for covered services in a policy period (usually a year). Once you reach this amount, your insurance plan pays 100% of the allowed amount for covered services.

Network

The network refers to the group of physicians, hospitals, and other healthcare providers that have agreed with your insurance company to provide services at a discounted rate. Staying within the network is a cornerstone of managing your healthcare costs effectively.

Pre-existing Condition

A pre-existing condition is any health issue that was diagnosed or treated before enrolling in a new health insurance plan. Historically, insurance plans could refuse coverage or charge higher rates for these conditions, but reforms have largely eliminated these practices, ensuring coverage for more individuals.

Explanation of Benefits (EOB)

The EOB isn't a bill but a document sent by your insurance company explaining what treatments and services were covered under your policy, the amount billed, payments made, and what you may owe to the provider. It's a crucial piece of the puzzle for understanding your healthcare expenses and ensuring that your bills are accurate.

Prior Authorization

Some services or medications require prior authorization, meaning your provider must get approval from your insurance company before the service is provided or the medication prescribed. This process ensures that the proposed service or medication is medically necessary and covered under your plan.

Understanding these terms and how they apply to different insurance policies is essential for navigating the healthcare system effectively. For medical billers, this knowledge is crucial in processing claims accurately, advising patients on their billing questions, and ensuring a smooth billing experience for all parties involved. By mastering the language of insurance, medical billers can serve as valuable intermediaries between healthcare providers, insurance companies, and patients, facilitating a better understanding and smoother process for everyone.

2.3 The Insurance Claim Process

Navigating the labyrinth of the insurance claim process is a pivotal skill for medical billers, akin to conducting a complex symphony where every note must be in perfect harmony. This process involves a series of meticulously orchestrated steps, ensuring that healthcare providers are reimbursed for their services while adhering to the myriad rules and regulations of insurance companies. Let's demystify this process, breaking it down into its core components and highlighting the critical role medical billers play at each stage.

Step 1: Patient Check-in and Verification of Insurance

The journey begins the moment a patient checks into a healthcare facility. Here, administrative staff collect the patient's insurance information and verify their coverage. This initial step is crucial; it sets the stage for the entire billing cycle. It involves confirming the patient's eligibility, understanding the specifics of their coverage, and identifying any potential issues that could lead to claim denial.

Step 2: Coding of Services

Once the healthcare service is provided, the next step is translating the details of the patient's visit into standardized codes. These codes are the universal language of medical billing, comprising CPT (Current Procedural Terminology) codes for procedures and ICD (International Classification of Diseases) codes for diagnoses. Accurate coding is essential, as it directly impacts the reimbursement process. This is where the medical biller's expertise in medical terminology and coding standards becomes invaluable.

Step 3: Creating and Submitting the Insurance Claim

Armed with the correct codes, the medical biller prepares the insurance claim. This document is a detailed invoice that includes the patient's information, the services provided, and the associated costs. The claim is then submitted to the insurance company, either electronically (the most common method today) or via paper forms. Timeliness and accuracy in this step are critical to avoid delays or denials.

Step 4: Insurance Company Processing

Upon receiving the claim, the insurance company undertakes its review process. This involves verifying the claim's accuracy, ensuring the services are covered under the patient's policy, and checking for any discrepancies that might flag the claim for denial. The insurance company may also conduct audits on certain claims to ensure compliance with their policies and procedures.

Step 5: Adjudication

Adjudication is the decision-making process where the insurance company determines the amount payable for the claim. This stage can result in the claim being fully paid, partially paid, denied, or rejected. Each outcome requires a different follow-up action from the medical biller, ranging from processing payments to addressing and appealing denials.

Step 6: Payment and Explanation of Benefits (EOB)

Once the claim is adjudicated, the insurance company issues payment to the healthcare provider, accompanied by an Explanation of Benefits (EOB). The EOB outlines the details of the payment, including what was covered, any deductibles or co-pays applied, and the reason for any denials. The medical biller reviews this document carefully to ensure that the payment matches the services provided.

Step 7: Patient Billing

The final step involves billing the patient for any remaining balance not covered by the insurance, such as deductibles, co-pays, or non-covered services. The medical biller prepares and sends an itemized bill to the patient, clearly explaining the charges and the payments made by the insurance company.

The Role of Medical Billers: Navigators of the Claim Process

Throughout this intricate process, medical billers act as navigators, ensuring that each step is executed with precision. Their role is not just administrative; it requires a deep understanding of healthcare services, insurance policies, and regulatory requirements. They must possess keen attention to detail, problem-solving skills, and the ability to communicate effectively with insurance companies, healthcare providers, and patients.

By mastering the insurance claim process, medical billers play a crucial role in the financial health of healthcare providers and ensure that patients can access the care they need without undue financial burden. This process, while complex, is essential for the smooth operation of the healthcare system, making the role of medical billers both challenging and profoundly important.

2.4 Exercise: 10 MCQs with Answers at the End

Test your understanding of navigating health insurance, including types of health insurance plans, key insurance terms and policies, and the insurance claim process with these multiple-choice questions. Find the correct answers provided at the end to check your comprehension.

Questions:

1. What type of health insurance plan requires members to select a primary care physician (PCP)?

   A) PPO

   B) HMO

   C) EPO

   D) HDHP

2. Which is a characteristic feature of a Preferred Provider Organization (PPO) plan?

   A) No out-of-network benefits

   B) Requires referrals to see specialists

   C) Flexibility to see doctors outside the network

   D) All services are provided within a closed network

3. What is a premium in health insurance?

   A) The amount paid for each service received

   B) The fixed amount paid before the insurance covers services

   C) The monthly cost to maintain the insurance policy

   D) The percentage of costs shared with the insurer after the deductible is met

4. A deductible is:

  A) A fixed fee for a specific service or medication

  B) The maximum amount an insured person pays out-of-pocket within a year

 C) An amount the insured must pay before insurance starts covering services

 D) The total cost of insurance per year

5. Co-insurance is best described as:

  A) A fixed amount paid for visiting specialists

  B) The amount paid annually for health coverage

  C) The percentage of costs shared by the insured and insurer after the deductible is met

  D) A set fee for prescription medications

6. The term "network" in health insurance refers to:

   A) The maximum amount that can be charged for covered services

   B) The group of healthcare providers contracted with the insurance company to provide services at negotiated rates

   C) A list of medications covered by the insurance plan

   D) The total number of policyholders within an insurance company

7. What does prior authorization mean in health insurance?

   A) Approval before a patient can enroll in an insurance plan

   B) Preliminary approval for a surgery by the primary care physician

   C) Pre-approval from the insurance company before receiving certain services or medications

   D) Authorization from a doctor before seeking emergency services

8. In the insurance claim process, adjudication refers to:

   A) The initial submission of a claim to the insurance company

   B) The verification of a patient's insurance coverage

   C) The decision-making process regarding the payment of a claim

   D) The final step where the patient is billed for services

9. An Explanation of Benefits (EOB) is:

   A) A detailed bill sent directly to the patient

   B) A document outlining the insurance company's payment decisions

   C) A summary of the patient's medical history

   D) A contract between the patient and the insurance provider

10. Which step is NOT directly involved in the insurance claim process?

   A) Coding of services

   B) Obtaining prior authorization

   C) Investing in health savings accounts (HSA)

   D) Patient check-in and verification of insurance

Answers:

1. B) HMO

2. C) Flexibility to see doctors outside the network

3. C) The monthly cost to maintain the insurance policy

4. C) An amount the insured must pay before insurance starts covering services

5. C) The percentage of costs shared by the insured and insurer after the deductible is met

6. B) The group of healthcare providers contracted with the insurance company to provide services at negotiated rates

7. C) Pre-approval from the insurance company before receiving certain services or medications

8. C) The decision-making process regarding the payment of a claim

9. B) A document outlining the insurance company's payment decisions

10. C) Investing in health savings accounts (HSA)

These questions and answers are designed to reinforce your understanding of key concepts related to health insurance that are crucial for medical billers and anyone navigating the healthcare system.

Chapter 3: Medical Coding Essentials

3.1 Introduction to Medical Coding

Embarking on the chapter of Medical Coding Essentials, we dive into the realm where healthcare meets the language of codes. Medical coding is a critical component of the healthcare system, serving as the universal language that translates complex medical procedures, diagnoses, and equipment into standardized codes. These codes are essential not only for billing and insurance purposes but also for maintaining patient records, tracking public health trends, and enhancing healthcare quality. Let's begin our journey into this fascinating and vital field with an introduction to medical coding.

The Foundation of Medical Coding

At its core, medical coding is about accuracy and precision. It's the process of converting everything from a routine doctor's visit to a complex surgical procedure into alphanumeric codes. These codes communicate critical information about medical conditions, treatments, and procedures in a concise and standardized format. This system enables healthcare providers to bill insurance companies accurately and efficiently, ensuring that patients receive the correct coverage for their treatments.

Why Is Medical Coding Important?

Medical coding goes beyond mere record-keeping and billing. It is instrumental in:

- **Ensuring Accurate Billing and Reimbursement:** Proper coding is essential for healthcare providers to receive timely and accurate payment for services rendered.

- **Facilitating Patient Care:** Accurate coding helps in creating a detailed and accessible patient history, which is vital for ongoing patient care, future treatments, and patient safety.

- **Supporting Public Health Research:** Aggregated coding data is used to track health trends, manage public health emergencies, and inform future healthcare policies.

- **Compliance and Reporting:** Coding plays a key role in compliance with healthcare regulations and in the reporting of healthcare data to government and regulatory bodies.

Key Coding Systems

There are several coding systems used in healthcare, each serving a specific purpose:

- **ICD (International Classification of Diseases):** This system is used to code diagnoses, symptoms, and procedures related to patient care. The ICD is critical for billing and epidemiological research, providing a uniform way to describe medical conditions across the globe.

- **CPT (Current Procedural Terminology):** Developed by the American Medical Association, CPT codes describe medical, surgical, and diagnostic services. They are crucial for outlining the services provided to patients and for insurance billing.

- **HCPCS (Healthcare Common Procedure Coding System):** HCPCS codes cover services and procedures not included in CPT, such as ambulance services and durable medical equipment. They play a significant role in billing Medicare and Medicaid.

The Role of Medical Coders

Medical coders are the skilled professionals behind the translation of medical records into codes. Their work requires a deep understanding of medical terminology, anatomy, and coding guidelines. Coders must stay up-to-date with coding changes and regulations to ensure compliance and accuracy. The role of a medical coder is both challenging and rewarding, offering a unique intersection between healthcare and data management.

Challenges in Medical Coding

Despite its systematic approach, medical coding faces several challenges, including keeping up with frequent updates to coding standards, managing complex cases, and ensuring accuracy in a fast-paced environment. Coders often work closely with healthcare providers to clarify diagnoses or treatments, ensuring that coding reflects the care delivered.

Conclusion

As we peel back the layers of medical coding, it's clear that this field is much more than assigning numbers to diagnoses and procedures. It's a critical component of the healthcare ecosystem, facilitating accurate billing, informed patient care, and the advancement of public health. As we delve deeper into the essentials of medical coding in the following sections, remember that at the heart of each code is a patient's story, making the role of medical coders both vital and profound.

3.2 Understanding CPT, ICD-10, and HCPCS

As we venture further into the world of medical coding, it becomes essential to understand the key coding systems that form the backbone of this intricate field. These systems, namely CPT (Current Procedural Terminology), ICD-10 (International Classification of Diseases, Tenth Revision), and HCPCS (Healthcare Common Procedure Coding System), serve distinct yet complementary roles in accurately documenting healthcare services and diagnoses. Let's explore each of these coding systems in detail, shedding light on their purposes, structures, and how they interplay in the medical billing process.

CPT (Current Procedural Terminology)

CPT codes are the cornerstone of billing for medical procedures and services. Developed and maintained by the American Medical Association (AMA), CPT codes provide a uniform language for describing medical, surgical, and diagnostic services. These codes ensure that healthcare providers, insurers, and patients speak a common language when discussing services rendered.

- **Structure:** CPT codes are five-digit numeric codes. They are organized into three categories:

  - **Category I:** Codes for widely used procedures and services, organized by body system or procedure type.

    - **Category II:** Supplemental tracking codes used for performance management.

    - **Category III:** Temporary codes for emerging technologies, services, and procedures.

CPT codes are updated annually, reflecting the latest advancements and trends in medical technology and procedures.

ICD-10 (International Classification of Diseases, Tenth Revision)

ICD-10 codes are a critical component of the healthcare coding system, providing a standardized classification for diagnoses and reasons for visits in all healthcare settings. Managed by the World Health Organization (WHO), ICD-10 codes allow for precise reporting of diseases, conditions, and signs and symptoms.

- **Structure:** ICD-10 codes can be alphanumeric and vary in length from 3 to 7 characters. The system is divided into:

  - **ICD-10-CM (Clinical Modification):** Used in all U.S. healthcare settings to code and classify morbidity data.

  - **ICD-10-PCS (Procedure Coding System):** Used in U.S. hospitals for inpatient procedures.

The transition to ICD-10 from its predecessor, ICD-9, expanded the number of available codes from around 14,000 to over 68,000, allowing for more specific and detailed reporting.

HCPCS (Healthcare Common Procedure Coding System)

HCPCS codes supplement CPT codes by covering services and products that may not be included in the CPT system, such as ambulance services, durable medical equipment, and certain drugs and biologicals. HCPCS is essential for billing Medicare and Medicaid services and is divided into two levels:

- **Level I:** Consists of the AMA's CPT codes.

- **Level II:** Alphanumeric codes that represent non-physician services, equipment, and supplies not covered by CPT.

HCPCS codes are updated annually to reflect the introduction of new services and technologies.

Interplay in Medical Billing

In the medical billing process, CPT and HCPCS codes are used to describe the procedures and services provided to a patient, while ICD-10 codes are used to detail the patient's diagnosis or reason for the service. This combination ensures a comprehensive billing statement that accurately reflects the care provided, facilitating appropriate reimbursement from payers.

Understanding and accurately applying CPT, ICD-10, and HCPCS codes are fundamental skills for medical coders. These coding systems not only ensure that healthcare providers are compensated for their services but also contribute to the broader goals of maintaining patient records, supporting public health initiatives, and ensuring the quality and continuity of care. As medical coding continues to evolve with healthcare advancements, the importance of mastering these coding systems becomes ever more critical for professionals in the field.

3.3 Common Coding Challenges

In the intricate world of medical coding, professionals often navigate a maze of challenges that require not only a deep understanding of coding systems but also an ability to adapt to the ever-changing landscape of healthcare regulations and practices. These challenges can impact the accuracy of billing, the efficiency of healthcare delivery, and ultimately, patient care. Here, we explore some of the common coding challenges and offer insights into overcoming them, ensuring both compliance and accuracy in medical documentation.

Keeping Up with Code Updates

Both CPT and ICD codes are subject to annual updates, which can include additions, deletions, and modifications. Staying abreast of these changes is crucial for coders to ensure that billing is accurate and compliant with current standards.

- **Solution:** Regular training and education, including webinars, workshops, and online courses, can help coders stay current. Subscribing to coding resources and publications from reputable organizations like the AMA and WHO also provides updates and insights.

Complexity of Coding Guidelines

Coding guidelines can be complex and nuanced, with specific rules that vary by code set and type of service. Misinterpretations or oversights can lead to incorrect coding, resulting in denials or delays in reimbursement.

- **Solution:** Coders should regularly review official coding guidelines and participate in coding forums or discussion groups to exchange knowledge and clarify doubts. Utilizing coding compliance software can also aid in ensuring adherence to guidelines.

Specificity of ICD-10 Codes

The specificity required by ICD-10 codes can be a double-edged sword. While it allows for detailed documentation of patient diagnoses, it also increases the potential for coding errors if documentation is not precise.

- **Solution:** Enhancing communication between coders and healthcare providers is key. Encouraging detailed and clear documentation from providers can help coders select the most accurate codes. Regular feedback loops between coders and clinicians can improve documentation practices over time.

Use of Electronic Health Records (EHRs)

While EHRs have revolutionized medical documentation, they also present challenges, such as template-based errors or copy-and-paste inaccuracies, leading to incorrect coding.

- **Solution:** Training on EHR best practices and the implementation of EHR audit tools can help identify and correct common mistakes. Coders should be trained to scrutinize EHR-generated documentation carefully to ensure accuracy before coding.

Dealing with Non-Specific Documentation

Sometimes, healthcare providers may document patient encounters with non-specific language that lacks the detail required for precise coding, especially in complex cases.

- **Solution:** Establishing a robust query process allows coders to request additional information from providers when documentation is unclear. Educating providers on the importance of specific, detailed documentation can also mitigate this issue.

Navigating Payer-Specific Rules

Insurance payers may have their own coding requirements or interpretations, which can vary significantly and affect the reimbursement process.

- **Solution:** Coders should familiarize themselves with payer-specific coding bulletins and guidelines. Building a reference library of payer-specific rules and regularly communicating with payer representatives can help clarify uncertainties.

Audits and Compliance

The threat of audits by regulatory bodies or insurance companies, aimed at uncovering coding inaccuracies and fraud, adds pressure to ensure coding compliance.

- **Solution:** Implementing regular internal or third-party audits can help identify and rectify coding issues before they become problematic. Investing in compliance and ethics training for coding staff reinforces the importance of accurate coding practices.

Conclusion

While the challenges in medical coding are significant, they are not insurmountable. Through continuous education, effective communication, and the use of technology, coders can navigate these hurdles successfully. Addressing these challenges head-on not only enhances the accuracy of medical billing but also contributes to the overall quality of healthcare delivery, ensuring that patients receive the care they need and providers are fairly compensated for their services.

3.4 Exercise: 10 MCQs with Answers at the End

Test your knowledge of medical coding essentials, including CPT, ICD-10, HCPCS, and common coding challenges with these multiple-choice questions. Evaluate your understanding and reinforce what you've learned in this chapter.

Questions:

1. Which coding system is used primarily for diagnostic coding in all healthcare settings?

   A) CPT

   B) ICD-10

C) HCPCS

D) EHR

2. CPT codes are updated:

A) Monthly

B) Quarterly

C) Annually

D) Biannually

3. HCPCS Level II codes are primarily used for:

A) Inpatient procedures

B) Physician services

C) Durable medical equipment and non-physician services

D) Diagnostic services

4. Which of the following best describes the purpose of ICD-10-PCS?

A) To code outpatient diagnoses

B) To code inpatient procedures

C) To code physician office visits

D) To code prescription medications

5. A major challenge in medical coding is:

A) The low volume of codes available

B) The static nature of coding guidelines

C) Keeping up with annual code updates

D) The simplicity of EHR systems

6. What is the primary solution for dealing with non-specific documentation?

A) Ignoring vague details

B) Establishing a robust query process

C) Using default codes

D) Requesting fewer details from healthcare providers

7. The specificity required by ICD-10 codes can lead to:

A) Easier coding processes

B) Reduced need for coder education

C) Increased potential for coding errors

D) Decreased healthcare costs

8. EHR template-based errors are an example of challenges related to:

A) Manual record keeping

B) Digital documentation systems

C) Outdated coding books

D) Healthcare provider training

9. Prioritizing continuous education for coders addresses which challenge?

A) Decreased healthcare demand

B) Keeping up with code updates and guidelines

C) Simplifying patient care procedures

D) Reducing the number of available codes

10. Payer-specific coding requirements affect:

A) The uniformity of coding practices

B) The need for coding audits

C) The reimbursement process

D) The annual update of CPT codes

Answers:

1. B) ICD-10

2. C) Annually

3. C) Durable medical equipment and non-physician services

4. B) To code inpatient procedures

5. C) Keeping up with annual code updates

6. B) Establishing a robust query process

7. C) Increased potential for coding errors

8. B) Digital documentation systems

9. B) Keeping up with code updates and guidelines

10. C) The reimbursement process

These questions are designed to help you solidify your understanding of medical coding essentials and the common challenges faced by coding professionals. Accurate and efficient coding is crucial for the healthcare industry, ensuring proper billing and contributing to the overall quality of patient care.

Chapter 4: The Billing Process

4.1 Patient Registration and Data Entry

The journey through the healthcare billing process begins at patient registration and data entry, a crucial phase that sets the foundation for accurate and efficient billing. This initial step involves collecting comprehensive patient information and entering it into the healthcare provider's system. It's akin to laying the groundwork for a building; if done correctly, it supports all subsequent steps, ensuring they proceed smoothly and efficiently. Let's delve into the intricacies of this foundational process and understand its significance in the billing cycle.

Patient Registration: The First Step

Patient registration is the patient's first interaction with the administrative side of healthcare. It's where the groundwork for the billing process is laid. During registration, patients provide essential information, including:

- **Personal Details:** Name, date of birth, address, and contact information.

- **Insurance Information:** Insurance provider, policy number, and group ID.

- **Medical History:** Previous conditions, allergies, current medications, and primary care physician.

This information not only aids in patient care but also in creating an accurate billing record. Ensuring the completeness and accuracy of this data is paramount, as errors or omissions can lead to claim denials or delays later in the billing process.

Data Entry: Digitizing Patient Information

Once collected, patient information is entered into the healthcare provider's electronic health record (EHR) system or practice management software. This step involves:

- **Digitizing Personal and Insurance Information:** Converting paper-based information into digital records.

- **Assigning Patient Identifiers:** Each patient is given a unique identifier to ensure that their medical and billing records are accurately linked and easily retrievable.

- **Verifying Insurance Details:** Checking the validity of the insurance information provided and understanding the coverage details to prepare for accurate billing.

Data entry must be performed with utmost accuracy. Mistakes made during this phase can propagate through the entire billing cycle, resulting in incorrect billing, insurance claim rejections, and potential delays in payment.

Importance of Accuracy and Verification

The significance of accuracy in patient registration and data entry cannot be overstated. Incorrect information can lead to a myriad of problems, including:

- **Claim Rejections:** Insurance companies may reject claims if there are discrepancies in patient information or if insurance details are outdated or incorrect.

- **Patient Dissatisfaction:** Errors in billing due to incorrect patient data can lead to patient frustration and dissatisfaction, impacting the provider's reputation.

- **Financial Delays:** Inaccuracies in registration and data entry can cause delays in payments to healthcare providers, affecting their financial stability.

To mitigate these issues, many healthcare providers implement verification processes, such as double-checking entered data against original documents and using software that flags incomplete or inconsistent information.

Leveraging Technology for Efficiency

Advancements in technology have significantly streamlined the patient registration and data entry process. Features like online pre-registration, electronic document management systems, and automated verification tools enhance accuracy and efficiency. These technologies not only reduce the administrative burden on staff but also improve the patient's experience by speeding up the check-in process and reducing wait times.

Conclusion

Patient registration and data entry are the bedrock of the healthcare billing process. The accuracy and thoroughness of these initial steps are crucial for the smooth operation of the entire billing cycle. By emphasizing accurate data collection, leveraging technology, and implementing robust verification processes, healthcare providers can ensure a seamless billing process that benefits both the provider and the patient. As we move forward in our exploration of the billing process, remember that the journey to accurate and efficient healthcare billing starts with the meticulous collection and entry of patient information.

4.2 Charge Entry and Claims Submission

After navigating the initial phase of patient registration and data entry, we transition to the critical steps of charge entry and claims submission within the healthcare billing process. This phase is where the services provided to the patient are translated into billable charges and meticulously prepared for submission to insurance payers. It's a delicate balance of precision and timeliness, requiring a deep understanding of coding systems and payer policies. Let's explore how medical billers convert healthcare services into claims and the importance of accuracy in this phase.

Charge Entry: The Art of Translating Care into Codes

Charge entry is the process of entering the data regarding the services provided, including procedures performed, into the billing software. Each service is assigned a specific code based on the CPT, ICD-10, and HCPCS coding systems, along with the appropriate charges. This step is crucial for several reasons:

- **Accuracy:** Correct charge entry ensures that claims are accurately represented for the services rendered, which is vital for receiving appropriate reimbursement.

- **Compliance:** It ensures compliance with coding guidelines and payer-specific billing rules, reducing the risk of audits and penalties.

- **Efficiency:** Accurate charge entry streamlines the billing process, reducing the need for claim resubmissions due to errors.

Key Components of Charge Entry

During charge entry, medical billers must pay close attention to several components, including:

- **Service Date and Location:** The date when and location where the service was provided, as this can affect reimbursement rates.

- **Provider Information:** Details of the healthcare provider who performed the service, necessary for claims processing.

- **Coding Accuracy:** Correct application of CPT, ICD-10, and HCPCS codes based on the documentation provided by the healthcare provider.

- **Modifiers:** Use of appropriate modifiers to accurately describe the services rendered, when necessary.

Claims Submission: Bridging Providers and Payers

Once charges are accurately entered, the next step is claims submission. This process involves sending the compiled claim, which now includes patient information, service codes, and charges, to the insurance payer. Claims can be submitted electronically through a clearinghouse or directly to the payer, depending on the requirements.

Challenges in Claims Submission

- **Timeliness:** Claims must be submitted within the payer-specific deadlines to be considered for reimbursement.

- **Payer Specifications:** Understanding and adhering to the unique submission guidelines of each insurance payer is essential.

- **Rejection and Denials:** Incorrectly filled claims can be rejected or denied, necessitating a thorough review and resubmission process.

Ensuring Successful Claims Submission

- **Verification of Information:** Double-checking patient information, codes, and charges for accuracy before submission.

- **Electronic Submission:** Utilizing electronic claims submission through a clearinghouse for efficiency and speed.

- **Follow-up:** Monitoring the status of submitted claims to quickly address any issues or denials.

The Importance of a Streamlined Process

Charge entry and claims submission are pivotal in the healthcare billing cycle. They require a detailed understanding of coding systems, payer policies, and billing practices. Streamlining these processes through training, technology, and clear communication can significantly impact a healthcare provider's financial health and patient satisfaction. By ensuring the accuracy and efficiency of charge entry and claims submission, medical billers play a vital role in the seamless operation of the healthcare billing system, facilitating timely reimbursements and minimizing financial discrepancies.

4.3 Payment Posting and Reconciliation

Following the meticulous steps of charge entry and claims submission, we reach the critical juncture of payment posting and reconciliation in the healthcare billing process. This phase is where payments received from insurance companies and patients are recorded, and the accuracy of these payments is verified against the billed charges. It's a phase that demands precision and attention to detail, as it directly impacts the financial integrity of healthcare providers and ensures that all services rendered are appropriately compensated.

Payment Posting: The Gateway to Financial Clarity

Payment posting involves the accurate recording of payments and adjustments to patient accounts within the billing system. It serves multiple purposes:

- **Financial Accuracy:** Ensures that the amounts paid by insurance companies and patients match the billed charges, highlighting discrepancies if any.

- **Revenue Tracking:** Helps in tracking the revenue flow of the healthcare provider, facilitating better financial planning and analysis.

- **Patient Account Management:** Updates patient accounts with payment information, aiding in the accurate calculation of outstanding balances.

Payments can be categorized into two types: payments from insurance companies (third-party payers) and payments directly from patients.

Challenges in Payment Posting

- **Complexity of EOBs/ERAs:** Explanation of Benefits (EOBs) from insurance companies and Electronic Remittance Advice (ERAs) can be complex, with multiple adjustments, denials, and partial payments that need to be accurately reflected in patient accounts.

- **Coordination with Multiple Payers:** Managing payments from various sources, including primary, secondary, and tertiary insurers, as well as patient payments, adds layers of complexity to the posting process.

Reconciliation: Ensuring Every Penny is Accounted For

Reconciliation is the process of comparing the posted payments and adjustments with the original billed amounts to identify any discrepancies. This step is vital for several reasons:

- **Accuracy in Financial Reporting:** It ensures that the healthcare provider's financial records accurately reflect the revenue received.

- **Identification of Underpayments and Denials:** Allows providers to identify and appeal underpayments or denied claims in a timely manner.

- **Compliance and Audit Readiness:** Maintains accurate and auditable financial records, crucial for compliance with healthcare regulations and readiness for potential audits.

Best Practices for Payment Posting and Reconciliation

- **Automated Posting Tools:** Utilizing automated payment posting tools can significantly reduce manual errors and increase efficiency by directly importing payment data from ERAs.

- **Regular Reconciliation Procedures:** Implementing regular, systematic reconciliation processes helps in early detection of discrepancies and underpayments.

- **Training and Education:** Ensuring that billing staff are well-trained in interpreting EOBs/ERAs and are familiar with the specific payment policies of major insurers.

- **Clear Communication:** Establishing clear channels of communication between the billing department and healthcare providers to resolve any discrepancies or questions regarding payment postings.

The Impact of Accurate Payment Posting and Reconciliation

Accurate payment posting and reconciliation are not merely administrative tasks; they are essential components of a healthy financial system for any healthcare provider. They ensure that services are compensated correctly, support the financial stability of providers, and maintain the trust of patients by ensuring transparent and accurate billing practices. As healthcare providers navigate the complexities of the billing process, prioritizing accuracy and efficiency in payment posting and reconciliation can lead to improved financial outcomes and enhanced patient satisfaction.

4.4 Exercise: 10 MCQs with Answers at the End

Test your understanding of the billing process, particularly focusing on patient registration and data entry, charge entry and claims submission, and payment posting and reconciliation, with these multiple-choice questions. Assess your grasp of these crucial steps in the healthcare billing cycle.

Questions:

1. What is the first step in the healthcare billing process?

   A) Charge Entry

   B) Claims Submission

   C) Patient Registration and Data Entry

   D) Payment Posting

2. CPT codes are used in which part of the billing process?

   A) Patient Registration

   B) Charge Entry

   C) Payment Posting

   D) Reconciliation

3. Which document is crucial for accurate payment posting?

   A) Patient Health Record

   B) Explanation of Benefits (EOB)

   C) Patient Registration Form

   D) Insurance Policy

4. What is the purpose of reconciliation in the billing process?

   A) To ensure patient information is accurate

   B) To verify payments against billed charges

   C) To submit claims to insurance

   D) To register new patients

5. Which of the following best describes charge entry?

   A) Recording patient personal details

   B) Submitting claims to insurance companies

   C) Translating healthcare services into billable charges

   D) Receiving payments from payers

6. Electronic submission of claims is part of which process?

   A) Patient Registration

   B) Charge Entry

C) Claims Submission

D) Payment Posting

7. The use of ICD-10 codes is crucial for which step?

A) Patient Registration

B) Charge Entry

C) Payment Posting

D) Reconciliation

8. Payment posting directly impacts:

A) The accuracy of patient medical records

B) The financial stability of the healthcare provider

C) The process of patient registration

D) The creation of new CPT codes

9. Regular, systematic reconciliation helps in:

A) Decreasing the number of patient visits

B) Early detection of underpayments and denials

C) Speeding up the patient registration process

D) Reducing the need for accurate charge entry

10. Accurate patient registration and data entry are essential for:

A) Ensuring the correct application of CPT codes

B) Facilitating timely claims submission

C) Directly receiving payments from patients

D) Preventing the need for reconciliation

Answers:

1. C) Patient Registration and Data Entry

2. B) Charge Entry

3. B) Explanation of Benefits (EOB)

4. B) To verify payments against billed charges

5. C) Translating healthcare services into billable charges

6. C) Claims Submission

7. B) Charge Entry

8. B) The financial stability of the healthcare provider

9. B) Early detection of underpayments and denials

10. B) Facilitating timely claims submission

These questions and answers are designed to reinforce your knowledge of the key components of the healthcare billing process, from the initial patient registration and data entry to the crucial steps of charge entry, claims submission, payment posting, and reconciliation. Understanding these processes is essential for ensuring accurate billing, timely reimbursement, and the overall financial health of healthcare providers.

Chapter 5: Legal and Regulatory Compliance

5.1 Healthcare Laws and Regulations

In the complex world of healthcare, adherence to legal and regulatory requirements is not just a matter of compliance but a fundamental aspect of providing quality care and maintaining trust. Healthcare laws and regulations are designed to protect patient rights, ensure the privacy and security of health information, and foster fair and accurate billing practices. This chapter delves into the crucial legal frameworks that govern the healthcare industry, emphasizing the importance of compliance for all stakeholders involved.

HIPAA: Ensuring Privacy and Security

The Health Insurance Portability and Accountability Act (HIPAA) of 1996 is a cornerstone of healthcare regulation, focusing on the protection of patient health information (PHI). HIPAA establishes standards for the privacy and security of PHI, impacting virtually all aspects of healthcare operations, from patient registration to billing processes.

- **Privacy Rule:** Sets standards for the use and disclosure of PHI, ensuring that patient information is shared only for legitimate purposes while allowing patients access to their own health records.

- **Security Rule:** Requires healthcare providers and their business associates to implement physical, administrative, and technical safeguards to protect electronic PHI (ePHI).

HITECH Act: Promoting Health Information Technology

The Health Information Technology for Economic and Clinical Health (HITECH) Act of 2009 builds on HIPAA's foundation, encouraging the adoption of electronic health records (EHR) and enhancing privacy and security protections for ePHI. It introduces stricter enforcement of HIPAA rules and increased penalties for breaches.

ACA: Expanding Access and Protecting Consumers

The Affordable Care Act (ACA) of 2010, among its many provisions, includes important protections for consumers, such as prohibiting insurance companies from denying coverage due to pre-existing conditions and extending coverage for young adults on their parents' plans. It also emphasizes the importance of preventive care and establishes the legal groundwork for healthcare exchanges.

False Claims Act: Preventing Fraud

The False Claims Act is a federal law that combats fraud against government programs, including Medicare and Medicaid. It allows for significant penalties against healthcare providers who knowingly submit false claims for government-funded services, emphasizing the importance of accurate billing and coding practices.

Stark Law and Anti-Kickback Statute: Preventing Conflicts of Interest

- **Stark Law:** Prohibits physicians from referring patients to entities with which they have a financial relationship for certain designated health services payable by Medicare or Medicaid, unless specific exceptions apply.

- **Anti-Kickback Statute:** Makes it illegal to knowingly and willfully offer, pay, solicit, or receive any remuneration to induce or reward referrals for services reimbursed by federal healthcare programs.

Compliance Programs: Mitigating Risks

To navigate the complex landscape of healthcare laws and regulations, healthcare providers implement comprehensive compliance programs. These programs typically include:

- **Policies and Procedures:** Developing clear guidelines that align with legal requirements.

- **Training and Education:** Regularly educating staff on compliance issues, legal obligations, and ethical standards.

- **Auditing and Monitoring:** Conducting regular reviews to ensure adherence to laws and internal policies.

- **Response and Prevention:** Establishing mechanisms to respond to compliance issues and prevent future violations.

Conclusion

Legal and regulatory compliance in healthcare is multifaceted, involving diligent adherence to laws and regulations that protect patients, ensure the integrity of health information, and promote fair billing practices. For healthcare providers, navigating this landscape requires a proactive approach, including continuous education, rigorous internal controls, and a commitment to ethical practices. As the healthcare industry evolves, staying informed about legal developments and adapting compliance strategies accordingly will be crucial for maintaining the trust and safety of patients and the public.

5.2 HIPAA Compliance

In the realm of healthcare, compliance with the Health Insurance Portability and Accountability Act (HIPAA) is not just a legal obligation but a critical component of patient trust and privacy protection. HIPAA, established in 1996, sets the standard for protecting sensitive patient information from being disclosed without the patient's consent or knowledge. Understanding and implementing HIPAA compliance is essential for all entities handling protected health information (PHI), including healthcare providers, insurance companies, and their business associates.

Key Provisions of HIPAA Compliance

HIPAA compliance revolves around several key provisions, each designed to safeguard patient privacy and the security of health information:

- **Privacy Rule:** This rule establishes national standards for the protection of PHI. It requires healthcare providers to take reasonable steps to ensure the privacy of patient communications and records. It also grants patients the right to access their health information, request corrections, and obtain a record of disclosures.

- **Security Rule:** The Security Rule sets standards for securing electronic protected health information (ePHI) by requiring physical, technical, and administrative safeguards. These include measures such as access controls, data encryption, and secure data transmission protocols to prevent unauthorized access to ePHI.

- **Breach Notification Rule:** This rule mandates that covered entities and their business associates notify individuals, the Department of Health and Human Services (HHS), and in some cases, the media, of any breach of unsecured PHI. Notifications must be made without unreasonable delay and no later than 60 days following the discovery of a breach.

- **Omnibus Rule:** The Omnibus Rule, enacted in 2013, strengthens the privacy and security protections established under HIPAA for individuals' health information, modifies the Breach Notification Rule, and extends the requirements to business associates of covered entities.

Implementing HIPAA Compliance

Achieving HIPAA compliance involves several steps and ongoing efforts to ensure that policies, procedures, and practices are in alignment with the regulations:

1. **Conduct a Risk Analysis:** Regularly perform a comprehensive risk analysis to identify potential vulnerabilities to the confidentiality, integrity, and availability of ePHI.

2. **Develop Policies and Procedures:** Establish clear, written policies and procedures that comply with HIPAA requirements, addressing the use, disclosure, and protection of PHI.

3. **Employee Training:** Provide regular training for all employees who handle PHI, ensuring they understand their roles and responsibilities under HIPAA.

4. **Implement Safeguards:** Apply appropriate physical, administrative, and technical safeguards to protect ePHI, including secure communication methods, encryption, and access controls.

5. **Manage Business Associates:** Ensure that all business associates who handle PHI on behalf of the entity comply with HIPAA requirements through Business Associate Agreements (BAAs).

6. **Incident Response and Reporting:** Develop and implement a process for responding to PHI breaches, including notification procedures in compliance with the Breach Notification Rule.

The Importance of HIPAA Compliance

Compliance with HIPAA is not merely a regulatory requirement; it is a foundational element of patient care and trust. By protecting patient privacy and securing health information, healthcare providers foster a safe environment where patients feel confident in sharing the information necessary for their care. Non-compliance with HIPAA can result in significant financial penalties, legal consequences, and damage to an organization's reputation.

In summary, HIPAA compliance is a continuous process that requires vigilance, dedication, and a culture of privacy and security within healthcare organizations. By adhering to HIPAA's regulations, healthcare providers and their associates not only fulfill their legal obligations but also contribute to the broader goal of enhancing patient care and protection in the healthcare ecosystem.

5.3 Fraud and Abuse in Medical Billing

Fraud and abuse in medical billing represent significant challenges within the healthcare system, impacting not only financial stability but also patient trust and the overall integrity of healthcare delivery. These unethical practices can lead to unnecessary costs for payers, including federal healthcare programs like Medicare and Medicaid, as well as private insurers, ultimately burdening taxpayers and policyholders. Understanding the nature of these practices, recognizing their signs, and implementing measures to prevent them are crucial steps in maintaining a fair, efficient, and trustworthy healthcare system.

Understanding Fraud and Abuse

- **Fraud** involves intentional deception or misrepresentation that an individual knows to be false or does not believe to be true, and makes, knowing that the deception could result in some unauthorized benefit to himself/herself or some other person. Examples include billing for services not rendered, falsifying a patient's diagnosis to justify unnecessary tests, and knowingly billing for services at a higher level than provided.

- **Abuse** refers to practices that, either directly or indirectly, result in unnecessary costs to the healthcare system. Abuse involves actions that may not involve intentional deception but are inconsistent with sound medical, business, or fiscal practices. Examples include billing for unnecessary medical services, charging excessively for services or supplies, and misusing codes on a claim, such as upcoding or unbundling codes.

Signs of Fraud and Abuse

Recognizing the signs of fraud and abuse is the first step in prevention. Key indicators include:

- Inconsistencies between patient records and billed services.

- Patterns of billing for the highest level of services in a category.

- Claims for services that are not usual for the patient's condition.

- Unusually high rates of certain procedures compared to peers.

Prevention and Compliance

Preventing fraud and abuse in medical billing requires a comprehensive approach, including:

1. **Education and Training:** Ensuring that all staff involved in billing and coding are aware of the regulations and ethical guidelines governing medical billing. Regular training sessions can help keep everyone updated on best practices and legal requirements.

2. **Implementation of Compliance Programs:** Developing and enforcing a compliance program that includes internal audits, monitoring, and procedures for reporting suspicious activities. A strong compliance program not only detects errors and violations but also deters unethical behavior.

3. **Use of Technology:** Leveraging technology, including software that flags potentially fraudulent or abusive billing patterns, can help in early detection and prevention. Automated systems can compare billing patterns against industry norms to identify outliers.

4. **Clear Reporting Mechanisms:** Establishing clear and confidential channels for reporting suspected fraud or abuse without fear of retaliation. Encouraging a culture of transparency and accountability is essential.

5. **Regular Audits and Reviews:** Conducting periodic audits of billing practices and procedures can identify and rectify issues before they escalate into serious legal problems.

Legal and Regulatory Framework

Several laws and regulations are designed to combat fraud and abuse in healthcare, including the False Claims Act (FCA), the Anti-Kickback Statute, and the Stark Law. Violations can result in significant penalties, including fines, exclusion from federal health programs, and even criminal charges.

The Role of Healthcare Providers

Healthcare providers play a crucial role in preventing fraud and abuse by adopting ethical billing practices, maintaining accurate and complete patient records, and ensuring that all claims accurately reflect the services provided. By fostering an organizational culture that prioritizes compliance and ethical practices, healthcare providers can help safeguard the integrity of the healthcare system.

Conclusion

Fraud and abuse in medical billing not only undermine the financial foundation of healthcare systems but also compromise the quality of patient care. Through vigilant prevention, education, and adherence to legal and ethical standards, healthcare providers and billing professionals can combat these practices, ensuring a more transparent, efficient, and trustworthy healthcare delivery system.

5.4 Exercise: 10 MCQs with Answers at the End

Test your understanding of legal and regulatory compliance in healthcare, focusing on healthcare laws and regulations, HIPAA compliance, and fraud and abuse in medical billing. These multiple-choice questions are designed to reinforce your knowledge and prepare you for practical application.

Questions:

1. What does HIPAA stand for?

   A) Health Insurance Probability and Accountability Act

   B) Health Insurance Portability and Accountability Act

   C) Healthcare Information Privacy and Assurance Act

   D) Healthcare Insurance Protection and Affordability Act

2. The HITECH Act is primarily concerned with:

A) Increasing health insurance coverage across the board

B) Promoting the adoption of electronic health records and enhancing privacy and security protections for healthcare information

C) Providing healthcare services to low-income families

D) Reducing healthcare fraud and abuse

3. Which law prohibits physicians from referring patients to services where they have a financial interest?

A) Anti-Kickback Statute

B) Stark Law

C) False Claims Act

D) Affordable Care Act

4. What is the primary purpose of the Breach Notification Rule under HIPAA?

A) To ensure that patients are notified of their rights under HIPAA

B) To mandate that healthcare providers notify patients when their PHI has been breached

C) To outline the procedures for transferring health insurance coverage

D) To define what constitutes a breach of electronic health information

5. Billing for services not rendered is an example of:

A) Abuse

B) Fraud

C) A Stark Law violation

D) A compliance program action

6. Which of the following best describes abuse in medical billing?

A) An intentional deception or misrepresentation for financial gain

B) Actions that result in unnecessary costs to healthcare programs, without direct evidence of intentional deception

C) Referring patients to a particular service for kickbacks

D) Violations of patient privacy under HIPAA

7. A compliance program for a healthcare provider typically includes:

A) Policies for patient care only

B) Training on office management systems

C) Measures for detecting and preventing fraud, waste, and abuse

D) Guidelines for choosing medical suppliers

8. The False Claims Act:

A) Encourages whistleblowers to report instances of fraud against government healthcare programs

B) Is focused solely on privacy breaches in healthcare settings

C) Deals with conflicts of interest in patient referrals

D) Governs the portability of health insurance coverage

9. Under HIPAA, when must covered entities notify individuals of a breach of unsecured PHI?

A) Within 30 days of discovery

B) Within 60 days of discovery

C) Within 90 days of discovery

D) Only if the breach affects more than 500 individuals

10. Which statement is true regarding the Anti-Kickback Statute?

A) It allows physicians to receive benefits for referring patients to certain services

B) It prohibits offering, paying, soliciting, or receiving remuneration to induce referrals for services covered by federal health programs

C) It is only applicable to the pharmaceutical industry

D) It was repealed by the Affordable Care Act

Answers:

1. B) Health Insurance Portability and Accountability Act

2. B) Promoting the adoption of electronic health records and enhancing privacy and security protections for healthcare information

3. B) Stark Law

4. B) To mandate that healthcare providers notify patients when their PHI has been breached

5. B) Fraud

6. B) Actions that result in unnecessary costs to healthcare programs, without direct evidence of intentional deception

7. C) Measures for detecting and preventing fraud, waste, and abuse

8. A) Encourages whistleblowers to report instances of fraud against government healthcare programs

9. B) Within 60 days of discovery

10. B) It prohibits offering, paying, soliciting, or receiving remuneration to induce referrals for services covered by federal health programs

These questions and answers are designed to deepen your understanding of the legal and regulatory aspects of healthcare compliance, emphasizing the importance of adhering to laws and regulations to ensure ethical practices, protect patient information, and prevent fraud and abuse in medical billing.

Chapter 6: Electronic Health Records (EHR)

6.1 Basics of EHR Systems

The transition from paper-based records to Electronic Health Records (EHR) systems represents one of the most significant advancements in modern healthcare. EHR systems offer a comprehensive, real-time view of patient health and history at the touch of a button, facilitating improved patient care, enhancing the efficiency of healthcare delivery, and paving the way for advancements in medical research. Understanding the basics of EHR systems is crucial for healthcare professionals navigating the digital transformation in healthcare.

What is an EHR System?

An Electronic Health Record (EHR) is a digital version of a patient's paper chart. EHRs are real-time, patient-centered records that make information available instantly and securely to authorized users. Unlike paper records, EHRs contain the medical and treatment histories of patients, allowing healthcare providers to access and share information with ease across different healthcare settings.

Key Features of EHR Systems

EHR systems come with a range of features designed to improve the quality and efficiency of healthcare, including:

- **Comprehensive Health Information:** EHRs include medical history, diagnoses, medications, treatment plans, immunization dates, allergies, radiology images, and laboratory test results.

- **Decision Support:** Many EHR systems offer clinical decision support tools to help providers make more informed care decisions.

- **Electronic Prescriptions:** EHRs can facilitate electronic prescribing, allowing healthcare providers to send prescriptions directly to pharmacies.

- **Patient Access:** Patients can access their health records, request prescription refills, and communicate with their healthcare providers through patient portals.

- **Data Reporting:** EHR systems can generate reports for managing clinical quality and for regulatory compliance purposes.

Benefits of EHR Systems

The adoption of EHR systems brings numerous benefits to healthcare providers, patients, and the healthcare system as a whole:

- **Improved Patient Care:** EHRs provide accurate, up-to-date, and complete information about patients at the point of care, enhancing the ability of healthcare providers to make well-informed treatment decisions.

- **Increased Efficiency:** EHRs reduce the need for paper records, minimize duplication of tests, and streamline workflows, saving time and resources.

- **Enhanced Coordination:** EHRs facilitate easier information sharing among healthcare providers, improving the coordination of care, especially for patients with complex conditions requiring care from multiple providers.

- **Better Patient Outcomes:** With comprehensive health information and clinical decision support, EHRs can contribute to better health outcomes through improved disease management and patient engagement.

- **Data Security:** EHR systems implement robust security measures to protect patient information, complying with HIPAA and other privacy regulations.

Challenges and Considerations

While EHR systems offer significant advantages, their implementation and use come with challenges, including:

- **Cost and Complexity:** The initial setup and ongoing maintenance of EHR systems can be costly and complex, particularly for smaller healthcare providers.

- **Training and Adoption:** Healthcare staff need comprehensive training to use EHR systems effectively, and there can be resistance to changing from traditional paper records.

- **Interoperability:** Sharing information across different EHR systems and healthcare settings remains a challenge, although standards and initiatives are in place to improve interoperability.

- **Privacy and Security:** Protecting the privacy and security of electronic health information is paramount, requiring ongoing vigilance and adherence to best practices.

Conclusion

EHR systems represent a foundational shift in the way healthcare is delivered and managed, offering the potential to significantly improve patient care, increase efficiency, and reduce costs. As technology evolves, the capabilities and benefits of EHRs are expected to expand, further transforming the healthcare landscape. Understanding the basics of EHR systems is essential for healthcare professionals to navigate this digital era, ensuring they can leverage these tools to provide the best possible care.

6.2 EHRs in Medical Billing

Electronic Health Records (EHRs) have revolutionized not just clinical care but also the financial aspects of healthcare, including medical billing. EHR systems streamline and integrate the billing process, offering a more efficient, accurate, and seamless way to manage patient charges and insurance claims. This integration has significant implications for revenue cycle management, reducing errors, and improving the overall financial health of healthcare practices.

Integration of Clinical and Billing Processes

One of the key advantages of EHR systems in medical billing is their ability to integrate clinical data directly with billing operations. This integration ensures that all billable services are accurately captured and coded, reducing the risk of lost charges or incorrect billing. Here's how EHRs impact various facets of the medical billing process:

- **Automated Charge Capture:** EHR systems automatically capture details of the care provided during a patient encounter, directly linking clinical services to billing codes. This automation reduces manual data entry and the potential for human error.

- **Enhanced Coding Accuracy:** With access to detailed patient records, billers can ensure that claims are coded accurately, reflecting the actual services provided. EHRs often include coding tools and alerts that help prevent common coding errors, such as undercoding or overcoding.

- **Streamlined Claims Submission:** EHR systems can generate and submit claims electronically to payers, speeding up the reimbursement process. They also facilitate real-time eligibility checks and pre-authorizations, reducing denials and delays.

- **Improved Documentation:** The comprehensive documentation within EHRs supports the billing process by providing detailed records of services rendered. This documentation is crucial for justifying claims to payers, especially in the case of audits or disputes.

Reducing Denials and Improving Cash Flow

EHRs play a significant role in reducing claim denials. By ensuring accurate and complete documentation, along with adherence to payer-specific billing rules, EHRs help minimize the common causes of denials. Furthermore, the ability to promptly address denied claims within the EHR system accelerates the resolution process, thereby improving cash flow.

Enhancing Patient Engagement and Transparency

EHRs also offer tools that enhance patient engagement with the billing process. Patient portals allow individuals to access their billing information, understand their financial responsibility, and make payments online. This transparency and convenience can lead to increased patient satisfaction and timely payments.

Challenges in Leveraging EHRs for Billing

Despite the benefits, there are challenges in fully leveraging EHR systems for billing, including:

- **Interoperability Issues:** Sharing billing information across different EHR systems and with payer systems can be challenging due to differences in data standards and formats.

- **Training and Adaptation:** Staff need comprehensive training to navigate EHR billing functionalities effectively. Adapting to new workflows requires time and may initially slow down the billing process.

- **Upfront Costs and Maintenance:** Implementing an EHR system with robust billing capabilities involves significant upfront costs and ongoing maintenance expenses.

Conclusion

EHRs in medical billing represent a paradigm shift towards more integrated, accurate, and efficient healthcare financial management. By bridging the gap between clinical care and billing, EHRs not only streamline revenue cycle management but also contribute to better patient care through improved accuracy and transparency. As technology advances, the potential for EHR systems to further enhance medical billing and financial operations in healthcare continues to grow, offering opportunities for practices to optimize their financial performance while maintaining high standards of patient care.

6.3 Data Security and Privacy

In the digital age, the security and privacy of electronic health records (EHRs) are paramount concerns for healthcare providers, patients, and regulatory bodies. As healthcare systems increasingly adopt EHRs, the vast amount of sensitive patient data stored and transmitted electronically has become a prime target for cyber threats. Ensuring data security and privacy is not just a regulatory requirement but a critical component of patient trust and care continuity. This section explores the challenges and strategies involved in safeguarding EHR data.

Challenges in EHR Data Security and Privacy

The digitization of health records presents several challenges that healthcare organizations must navigate to protect patient information:

- **Cybersecurity Threats:** Healthcare data is highly valuable on the black market, making EHR systems a target for hackers. Threats include ransomware, phishing attacks, and data breaches.

- **Insider Threats:** Not all threats are external. Insider threats, whether through malicious intent or accidental breaches, pose significant risks to data security.

- **Complex Regulatory Environment:** Compliance with laws like HIPAA in the US, GDPR in Europe, and other regional data protection regulations adds layers of complexity to data security and privacy practices.

- **Interoperability and Data Sharing:** As healthcare providers share patient data across platforms and organizations to improve care coordination, ensuring the security of data in transit and at rest becomes increasingly challenging.

Strategies for Enhancing EHR Data Security and Privacy

To address these challenges, healthcare organizations implement a multifaceted approach to data security and privacy:

- **Encryption:** Encrypting data both at rest and in transit ensures that even if data is intercepted or accessed by unauthorized individuals, it remains unreadable and secure.

- **Access Controls:** Implementing stringent access controls and authentication measures, such as multi-factor authentication (MFA), ensures that only authorized personnel can access sensitive patient information.

- **Regular Audits and Monitoring:** Conducting regular security audits and continuously monitoring EHR systems for unusual activities can help detect and mitigate potential threats early.

- **Employee Training:** Since human error can lead to data breaches, regular training for all staff members on data security best practices and awareness of phishing and other cyber threats is crucial.

- **Data Backup and Disaster Recovery Plans:** Regularly backing up EHR data and having a robust disaster recovery plan in place ensure that patient information can be restored and accessed even after a cybersecurity incident or natural disaster.

- **Compliance with Legal Standards:** Adhering to HIPAA and other relevant data protection regulations by implementing policies and procedures for the use, disclosure, and protection of patient information is mandatory for avoiding legal penalties and maintaining patient trust.

The Role of Patients in Data Security

Empowering patients to be active participants in their healthcare data security is also essential. This involves:

- Providing patients with access to their health records through secure patient portals.

- Educating patients on the importance of data privacy and security, including how to recognize phishing attempts and secure their personal information.

- Offering options for patients to control the sharing of their health information.

Conclusion

The security and privacy of EHR data are critical to the integrity of healthcare delivery and the protection of patient rights. By employing comprehensive security measures, conducting regular training, and fostering a culture of privacy and security awareness, healthcare organizations can better protect against the evolving landscape of cyber threats. As technology advances, the commitment to safeguarding the confidentiality, integrity, and availability of electronic health information must remain a top priority for all stakeholders in the healthcare ecosystem.

6.4 Exercise: 10 MCQs with Answers at the End

Test your knowledge on the topics of Electronic Health Records (EHRs), focusing on the basics, their role in medical billing, and the crucial aspects of data security and privacy. This exercise will help reinforce your understanding and ensure you grasp the key concepts and applications of EHR systems in modern healthcare.

Questions:

1. What is the primary purpose of an EHR system?

   A) To automate appointment scheduling

   B) To provide a digital version of a patient's medical history

   C) To manage hospital inventory

   D) To secure email communications within a healthcare facility

2. Which feature is commonly found in EHR systems?

   A) Automatic billing

   B) Clinical decision support

   C) Online marketing tools

   D) Inventory tracking

3. What does the HITECH Act primarily promote?

   A) The use of telemedicine

   B) The adoption of electronic health records and enhancing their privacy and security

   C) The development of new pharmaceuticals

   D) Reduction in healthcare staffing

4. What is a significant benefit of EHRs in medical billing?

   A) Decreasing the need for patient consent

   B) Automated charge capture and enhanced coding accuracy

   C) Eliminating the need for insurance

   D) Reducing patient interaction with providers

5. Which of the following is a key challenge in EHR data security?

A) Overstaffing in healthcare IT departments

B) Cybersecurity threats

C) Excessive data storage capacity

D) Lack of data to analyze

6. The HIPAA Privacy Rule is designed to:

A) Prevent the sharing of any healthcare information

B) Protect the privacy of individual health information

C) Discourage the use of electronic health records

D) Promote the sharing of health data without consent

7. An effective strategy for enhancing EHR data security is:

A) Using simple passwords for ease of access

B) Encryption of data both at rest and in transit

C) Limiting data backup frequency

D) Sharing passwords among medical staff for convenience

8. What role do patients have in their healthcare data security with EHR systems?

A) They have no role or responsibility

B) Monitoring healthcare provider's security measures

C) Accessing their health records through secure portals

D) Developing and implementing security protocols for their data

9. Regular training for staff on data security best practices is crucial to prevent:

A) Financial overinvestment in technology

B) Cybersecurity threats and human error

C) Patients from accessing their own data

D) The use of electronic health records altogether

10. Which law requires covered entities to notify individuals of a breach of unsecured PHI?

A) The Affordable Care Act

B) The Anti-Kickback Statute

C) The HIPAA Breach Notification Rule

D) The Stark Law

Answers:

1. B) To provide a digital version of a patient's medical history

2. B) Clinical decision support

3. B) The adoption of electronic health records and enhancing their privacy and security

4. B) Automated charge capture and enhanced coding accuracy

5. B) Cybersecurity threats

6. B) Protect the privacy of individual health information

7. B) Encryption of data both at rest and in transit

8. C) Accessing their health records through secure portals

9. B) Cybersecurity threats and human error

10. C) The HIPAA Breach Notification Rule

These questions and answers are designed to solidify your comprehension of the critical aspects of EHR systems, from their implementation and impact on medical billing to the paramount importance of ensuring data security and privacy.

Chapter 7: Advanced Coding Techniques

7.1 Specialized Coding Strategies

As the healthcare industry evolves, so does the complexity of medical coding. Advanced coding techniques and specialized strategies are essential for accurately capturing the full scope of healthcare services provided. These advanced approaches not only ensure compliance with ever-changing regulations but also maximize reimbursement and minimize denials. This section explores several specialized coding strategies that are crucial for navigating the complexities of modern healthcare billing.

1. Hierarchical Condition Categories (HCC) Coding

HCC coding is a risk adjustment model used primarily in Medicare Advantage and other payer programs to predict future healthcare costs based on the diagnosis codes submitted. This model emphasizes the importance of coding chronic conditions accurately and completely every year. HCC coding requires a deep understanding of disease processes and documentation practices to capture all relevant diagnoses that affect patient risk scores.

Strategies for Effective HCC Coding:

- **Comprehensive Review:** Regularly review patient records for chronic conditions that may have been previously documented but not coded in the current year.

- **Continuous Education:** Stay updated on changes to HCC categories and guidelines through continuous education and training.

2. Quality Measure Coding

Quality measure coding involves capturing data that reflects the quality of care provided, which is increasingly used by payers to determine reimbursement rates and bonuses. This coding focuses on preventive measures, management of chronic diseases, and outcomes.

Strategies for Optimizing Quality Measure Coding:

- **Proactive Documentation:** Work closely with healthcare providers to ensure that services meeting quality measures are documented thoroughly.

- **Regular Audits:** Conduct audits to identify missed opportunities for capturing quality measures in coding.

3. Use of Modifiers

Modifiers play a critical role in coding by providing additional information about services rendered without changing the meaning of the code itself. Proper use of modifiers can prevent denials for seemingly duplicate services or procedures that are part of a more extensive treatment.

Strategies for Accurate Use of Modifiers:

- **Detailed Knowledge:** Understand the specific requirements for common modifiers and when their use is justified.

- **Provider Education:** Educate providers on the necessity of detailed documentation to support the use of modifiers.

4. Specialty-Specific Coding

Medical specialties often have unique coding challenges and opportunities. Specialty-specific coding requires an in-depth understanding of the procedures, services, and common diagnoses within a particular specialty.

Strategies for Specialty-Specific Coding:

- **Specialized Training:** Invest in specialty-specific training and resources to understand the nuances of coding for different medical specialties.

- **Collaboration:** Work closely with providers in the specialty to understand the specifics of procedures and services offered.

5. Advanced E/M Coding

With the updates to Evaluation and Management (E/M) coding guidelines, coders must adapt to new ways of determining the level of service based on either time or medical decision-making.

Strategies for Adapting to E/M Coding Changes:

- **Thorough Review of Guidelines:** Regularly review and understand the updated E/M coding guidelines.

- **Provider Training:** Assist providers in understanding how their documentation practices need to change to meet the new E/M coding requirements.

Conclusion

Advanced coding techniques require a proactive approach, continuous education, and a collaborative effort between coders and healthcare providers. By employing specialized coding strategies, medical coders can ensure that they accurately capture the complexity of the care provided, leading to appropriate reimbursement and supporting the financial health of healthcare organizations.

7.2 Coding for Complex Cases

Coding for complex cases in medical billing presents a unique set of challenges that require advanced knowledge, precision, and a strategic approach. Complex cases often involve multiple diagnoses, intricate procedures, or conditions that affect coding and billing processes significantly. Navigating these complexities efficiently is crucial for ensuring accurate reimbursement and compliance with healthcare regulations. This section explores key considerations and strategies for coding complex cases.

Understanding the Complexity

Complex cases may include chronic conditions with exacerbations, multiple injuries from a single incident, or patients undergoing numerous treatments and procedures during one hospital stay. These scenarios demand a nuanced understanding of coding guidelines to accurately represent the patient's condition and the care provided.

Key Considerations for Coding Complex Cases

1. **Comprehensive Documentation:** The foundation for accurate coding lies in detailed and precise documentation by healthcare providers. Coders rely on this documentation to identify all relevant diagnoses and procedures for coding.

2. **Hierarchical Coding:** Certain conditions and treatments have coding hierarchies that must be followed. Understanding the order in which diagnoses should be coded, based on their relevance and impact on patient care, is essential.

3. **Chronic Conditions and Comorbidities:** Chronic conditions and comorbidities can complicate the coding process, especially when they influence the care provided. Coders must ensure that such conditions are accurately captured and coded, as they can affect risk adjustment and reimbursement.

4. **Procedure Combinations:** Some complex cases involve procedures that are performed together or influence each other. Coders must be aware of bundling rules and guidelines for coding multiple procedures to avoid denials or underbilling.

Strategies for Success

1. **Continuous Education:** Stay updated on coding guidelines, payer policies, and industry best practices through ongoing education and training. Specialized seminars and coding resources for complex cases can provide valuable insights.

2. **Use of Advanced Coding Tools:** Leverage coding software and tools that offer guidance on complex coding scenarios, including hierarchical condition categories (HCC) and the latest ICD, CPT, and HCPCS codes.

3. **Query Process:** Implement an effective query process to clarify ambiguous or incomplete documentation with healthcare providers. Clear communication can resolve uncertainties and ensure accurate coding.

4. **Peer Review:** For highly complex cases, peer review among coding professionals can help identify potential errors or omissions before submission. Collaborative approaches foster accuracy and compliance.

5. **Specialized Focus:** Consider developing expertise in coding for specific complex conditions or treatments. Specialized knowledge can improve accuracy and efficiency in handling similar cases.

6. **Auditing and Quality Assurance:** Regular audits of coded complex cases can identify patterns of errors or areas for improvement. Feedback from these audits contributes to continuous learning and coding accuracy.

Conclusion

Coding for complex cases requires a blend of detailed knowledge, strategic thinking, and collaboration with clinical staff. By focusing on comprehensive documentation, understanding coding hierarchies, and employing strategic coding practices, coders can navigate the challenges of complex cases effectively. This not only ensures accurate reimbursement but also supports the overall goal of delivering quality patient care.

7.3 Updates in Medical Coding

The field of medical coding is dynamic, with regular updates to coding standards, guidelines, and reimbursement policies to reflect advances in medical science, changes in healthcare delivery, and shifts in regulatory and payer requirements. Staying abreast of these updates is crucial for medical coders, billing professionals, and healthcare providers to ensure accurate billing, compliance, and optimized reimbursement. This section outlines the importance of keeping up with coding updates and strategies for doing so effectively.

Why Medical Coding Updates Are Critical

1. **Accuracy and Compliance:** Coding updates often include new codes, revisions, deletions, and changes to coding guidelines. These updates are essential for accurately reflecting current medical practices and ensuring compliance with healthcare regulations and payer policies.

2. **Reimbursement:** Accurate and up-to-date coding directly impacts the reimbursement process. Using outdated codes can lead to claim denials, delays, and the need for re-submission, affecting the financial health of healthcare practices.

3. **Quality of Care:** Coding updates reflect new technologies, treatments, and procedures that can improve patient care. By using the latest codes, healthcare providers can accurately document and bill for cutting-edge services.

Sources of Coding Updates

- **ICD (International Classification of Diseases):** Updated by the World Health Organization (WHO) and adapted by national authorities (e.g., ICD-10-CM in the United States by the CDC).

- **CPT (Current Procedural Terminology):** Updated annually by the American Medical Association (AMA).

- **HCPCS (Healthcare Common Procedure Coding System):** Updated annually by the Centers for Medicare & Medicaid Services (CMS).

- **Specialty-specific coding guidelines:** Updated by professional associations and specialty societies.

Strategies for Staying Updated

1. **Continuing Education:** Participate in continuing education programs, workshops, webinars, and conferences focused on medical coding. Many professional associations offer these resources.

2. **Professional Associations:** Membership in professional associations like the American Health Information Management

Association (AHIMA) or the American Academy of Professional Coders (AAPC) provides access to a wealth of resources, including coding updates, newsletters, and journals.

3. **Online Resources and Social Media:** Leverage online platforms, forums, and social media groups dedicated to medical coding. These can be valuable sources of real-time information and peer support.

4. **Coding Software and Tools:** Use coding software and tools that receive regular updates to incorporate the latest coding standards and guidelines.

5. **Internal Communication:** Establish a system within your organization for disseminating coding updates. Regular meetings, emails, or an internal online forum can help ensure that all coding and billing staff are informed of the latest changes.

6. **Feedback Loop:** Create a feedback loop with clinicians to discuss documentation practices in light of coding updates. This collaboration can help improve the accuracy of medical records and coding.

Challenges in Keeping Up with Updates

- **Volume of Changes:** The sheer volume of updates can be overwhelming, particularly when they involve significant changes to coding systems or guidelines.

- **Resource Constraints:** Small practices may lack the resources for extensive training and subscriptions to all relevant publications and software updates.

Conclusion

Staying informed about updates in medical coding is a continuous and essential process for coding professionals. By employing effective strategies for education, utilizing resources from professional associations, and leveraging technology, coders can navigate the complexities of coding updates. This commitment to staying informed not only enhances coding accuracy and compliance but also supports the overall mission of delivering high-quality patient care.

7.4 Exercise: 10 MCQs with Answers at the End

Test your knowledge of advanced coding techniques, including specialized coding strategies, handling complex cases, and staying updated with medical coding changes. This exercise is designed to reinforce your understanding of these critical aspects in the evolving field of medical coding.

Questions:

1. Hierarchical Condition Categories (HCC) coding is crucial for:

   A) Predicting hospital inventory needs.

   B) Adjusting patient risk scores and predicting future healthcare costs.

   C) Documenting outpatient procedures only.

   D) Simplifying the medical billing process for primary care.

2. Quality measure coding affects reimbursement by:

   A) Reducing the overall number of codes used.

   B) Highlighting the efficiency of the billing department.

   C) Reflecting the quality of care provided, influencing reimbursement rates.

   D) Decreasing the time needed for claim processing.

3. The use of modifiers in medical coding:

   A) Is optional and rarely impacts reimbursement.

   B) Can prevent denials for seemingly duplicate services.

   C) Simplifies the coding process by reducing the number of codes needed.

D) Is primarily used for cosmetic procedures.

4. A significant benefit of specialty-specific coding is:

A) It eliminates the need for general medical knowledge.

B) Reduces the importance of coding accuracy.

C) Improves coding accuracy and efficiency for specific medical specialties.

D) Allows the use of a universal coding system across all specialties.

5. Updates to Evaluation and Management (E/M) coding guidelines:

A) Are made daily to keep coders alert.

B) Have simplified documentation requirements for coding based on time or medical decision-making.

C) Require less detailed patient information for billing purposes.

D) Eliminate the need for coding training and education.

6. A challenge in staying updated with medical coding is:

A) The limited number of updates that occur.

B) The predictability and consistency of changes.

C) The volume of changes and resource constraints for training.

D) The decreased importance of coding in modern healthcare.

7. Continuous education for medical coders:

A) Is only necessary for beginners in the field.

B) Can include webinars, workshops, and professional association resources.

C) Should be avoided to prevent information overload.

D) Focuses exclusively on manual coding techniques.

8. The primary purpose of coding audits and quality assurance is to:

A) Punish coders for mistakes.

B) Identify patterns of errors or areas for improvement.

C) Reduce the workload of medical coders.

D) Phase out the use of ICD codes.

9. Effective strategies for coding complex cases include:

A) Ignoring less significant secondary diagnoses.

B) Utilizing advanced coding tools and conducting regular audits.

C) Focusing solely on the primary diagnosis for simplicity.

D) Limiting communication with healthcare providers to reduce confusion.

10. The adoption of electronic health records (EHRs) impacts medical coding by:

   A) Decreasing the accuracy of patient health information.

   B) Increasing the reliance on paper documentation.

   C) Enhancing the integration of clinical data with billing operations.

   D) Simplifying legal compliance to a minimal level.

Answers:

1. B) Adjusting patient risk scores and predicting future healthcare costs.

2. C) Reflecting the quality of care provided, influencing reimbursement rates.

3. B) Can prevent denials for seemingly duplicate services.

4. C) Improves coding accuracy and efficiency for specific medical specialties.

5. B) Have simplified documentation requirements for coding based on time or medical decision-making.

6. C) The volume of changes and resource constraints for training.

7. B) Can include webinars, workshops, and professional association resources.

8. B) Identify patterns of errors or areas for improvement.

9. B) Utilizing advanced coding tools and conducting regular audits.

10. C) Enhancing the integration of clinical data with billing operations.

These questions and answers aim to solidify your understanding of advanced medical coding techniques and the continuous need for education and adaptation in the field.

Chapter 8: Insurance Claim Denials and Appeals

8.1 Understanding Claim Denials

Navigating the intricacies of insurance claim denials is a critical aspect of medical billing and revenue cycle management. A claim denial occurs when an insurance company refuses to pay for healthcare services rendered, citing various reasons that can range from administrative errors to policy exclusions. Understanding why claims are denied and how to address these denials is essential for maintaining financial health and ensuring that healthcare providers are compensated for their services.

Types of Claim Denials

Claim denials can be broadly categorized into two types: **soft denials** and **hard denials**.

- **Soft Denials:** These are temporary denials with the potential for payment after additional information is provided or specific issues are corrected. Examples include denials due to missing information or verification needs.

- **Hard Denials:** These result in lost or written-off revenue unless successfully appealed. Hard denials often involve issues like non-covered services, policy exclusions, or coding errors that violate payer contract terms.

Common Reasons for Claim Denials

1. **Incomplete or Incorrect Information:** Simple mistakes such as misspelled patient names, incorrect policy numbers, or missing codes can lead to denials.

2. **Lack of Authorization or Pre-Certification:** Failing to obtain the necessary pre-authorization for procedures or not adhering to referral requirements.

3. **Service Not Covered:** The service provided is not covered under the patient's insurance plan or is deemed not medically necessary.

4. **Coding Errors:** Incorrect, incomplete, or outdated coding can result in denials, emphasizing the importance of accurate medical coding.

5. **Timely Filing Exceeded:** Claims submitted after the insurance company's deadline can be denied for late filing.

Strategies for Minimizing Claim Denials

- **Thorough Verification Process:** Implement a robust verification process to ensure all patient and insurance information is accurate and complete before submitting claims.

- **Stay Updated on Coding and Billing Practices:** Regular training and updates on the latest coding practices and payer guidelines can help reduce coding-related denials.

- **Pre-Authorization and Pre-Certification:** Always verify the need for pre-authorization or pre-certification for procedures and obtain them in advance.

- **Timely Submission:** Develop a system to ensure all claims are submitted within the payer's filing deadlines.

- **Clear Documentation:** Ensure that all services are well-documented and that the documentation supports the necessity of the care provided.

The Appeals Process

When a claim is denied, healthcare providers have the right to appeal the decision. The appeals process involves reviewing the denial, gathering necessary documentation and information, and submitting a formal appeal to the insurance company.

Understanding the specific reason for the denial and addressing it directly in the appeal is crucial for success.

Conclusion

Understanding and effectively managing claim denials are vital skills in medical billing. By identifying common reasons for denials and implementing strategies to address them, healthcare providers can improve their billing practices, reduce the number of denials, and ensure timely and appropriate reimbursement for services rendered. In cases where denials occur, knowing how to navigate the appeals process can recover revenue that would otherwise be lost.

8.2 Effective Appeal Strategies

When an insurance claim is denied, it's not necessarily the end of the road. An effective appeal can often reverse the decision, securing reimbursement for services provided. Understanding how to construct a compelling appeal is crucial for healthcare providers to challenge unjust denials successfully. This involves a clear understanding of the denial reason, meticulous preparation of supporting documentation, and adherence to the insurer's appeal process.

Steps for Constructing an Effective Appeal

1. **Review the Denial Notice:** Carefully read the explanation of benefits (EOB) or the denial letter to understand the specific reasons for the denial. This information is crucial for crafting your appeal strategy.

2. **Understand the Policy:** Review the patient's insurance policy to understand the coverage details and the insurer's reasons for considering the claim non-payable. This review can often reveal if the denial was due to an oversight or misunderstanding of the policy terms.

3. **Gather Supporting Documentation:** Collect all relevant documentation that supports the necessity and appropriateness of the care provided. This might include medical records, physician notes, test results, and a detailed letter of medical necessity.

4. **Check for Errors:** Re-examine the claim for any possible coding or billing errors. Simple mistakes such as incorrect patient information, coding errors, or missing documentation can often be the cause of denials.

5. **Write a Concise Appeal Letter:** Prepare a clear and concise appeal letter that outlines the reasons why the denial should be reconsidered. Include references to specific policy provisions, medical guidelines, or coding standards that support your case.

6. **Follow the Insurer's Appeal Process:** Each insurance company has its own procedures for filing an appeal. Ensure that you follow these guidelines carefully, including deadlines for submitting an appeal and any specific forms or documentation required.

Tips for a Successful Appeal

- **Be Timely:** Pay close attention to the appeal submission deadlines. Submitting an appeal as soon as possible, while ensuring that all necessary documentation is included, can prevent further delays.

- **Stay Organized:** Keep detailed records of all communications with the insurance company, including dates of conversations, names of representatives, and the specifics of what was discussed.

- **Be Persistent:** If the first appeal is denied, you may have the option to escalate the appeal to a higher level within the insurance company or to an external review board.

- **Seek Expert Advice:** Consider consulting with a healthcare attorney or a billing specialist with experience in appeals for complex cases or significant amounts.

- **Patient Involvement:** In some cases, involving the patient can be beneficial, especially if they can provide additional information or if their policy allows them to initiate an appeal directly.

Conclusion

Navigating the appeals process requires patience, precision, and a thorough understanding of healthcare billing practices and insurance policies. By employing effective appeal strategies, healthcare providers can advocate for rightful reimbursement, ensuring that they are compensated for the care provided. Success in the appeals process not only impacts the financial health of the practice but also reinforces the commitment to patient care by striving to resolve coverage issues that may affect treatment access.

8.3 Managing Patient Communications

Effectively managing patient communications during the insurance claim denial and appeals process is critical for maintaining trust and transparency with patients. When a claim is denied, patients may feel anxious, confused, or frustrated, fearing the financial burden of uncovered medical expenses. Healthcare providers have a responsibility to navigate these situations with care, ensuring patients are informed, supported, and involved in the resolution process. This section outlines strategies for managing patient communications effectively during these challenging times.

Clear Explanation of the Denial

1. **Initial Notification:** Promptly inform the patient of the denial, using clear and understandable language. Explain the specific reason for the denial as provided by the insurance company.

2. **Written Communication:** Follow up with a written explanation, including a copy of the denial notice and a clear explanation of what it means. This helps ensure that the patient fully understands the situation and has a record of the communication.

Guidance on Next Steps

1. **Appeal Process:** Explain the appeal process, including the steps you, as the healthcare provider, will take to appeal the denial on their behalf. Offer guidance on how patients can participate in the appeal process if appropriate.

2. **Patient Responsibilities:** Clearly outline any actions the patient may need to take, such as providing additional information, contacting their insurance company, or considering alternative payment arrangements.

3. **Timeline and Expectations:** Provide a realistic timeline for the appeal process and set expectations regarding possible

outcomes. Ensure patients understand that while you are advocating on their behalf, the final decision rests with the insurance company.

Support and Reassurance

1. **Empathy:** Show empathy and understanding for the patient's concerns. A claim denial can be distressing, and patients need to feel supported throughout the process.

2. **Accessibility:** Ensure patients know how to contact your office with questions or concerns about their denied claim. Provide a specific point of contact for streamlined communication.

3. **Financial Counseling:** Offer financial counseling services to help patients understand their options, including payment plans, financial assistance programs, or alternative insurance solutions.

Patient Advocacy

1. **Advocate for the Patient:** Demonstrate your commitment to advocating for your patients by vigorously pursuing the appeal process and exploring all avenues to overturn the denial.

2. **Transparency:** Keep patients informed about the progress of the appeal, including any setbacks or advancements. Regular

updates help maintain trust and reassure patients that their case is being actively managed.

3. **Educational Resources:** Provide patients with resources or direct them to advocacy groups that can offer additional support and guidance on dealing with insurance denials and appeals.

Conclusion

Effective communication with patients during the claim denial and appeals process is fundamental to maintaining a positive patient-provider relationship. By providing clear explanations, guidance, and support, healthcare providers can help mitigate the stress and uncertainty associated with insurance denials. Moreover, demonstrating a commitment to patient advocacy strengthens trust and can positively impact patient satisfaction and loyalty.

8.4 Exercise: 10 MCQs with Answers at the End

Test your understanding of insurance claim denials and appeals, focusing on the processes involved, effective appeal strategies, and best practices for managing patient communications. This exercise aims to reinforce key concepts and prepare you for handling these scenarios in a healthcare setting.

Questions:

1. What is a common reason for insurance claim denials?

   A) Patient satisfaction with the service provided

   B) Lack of pre-authorization for a procedure

   C) Overpayment for previous services

   D) Patient opting for alternative treatment methods

2. A "soft denial" can be described as:

   A) A permanent refusal to pay a claim

   B) A denial that cannot be appealed

   C) A temporary denial that may be reversed upon submission of additional information

   D) A denial issued without a specific reason

3. Effective strategies for appealing a claim denial include:

   A) Waiting for the patient to contact the insurance company

   B) Ignoring the denial notice and resubmitting the same claim

   C) Gathering supporting documentation and writing a concise appeal letter

   D) Advising the patient to pay the bill in full to avoid hassle

4. When managing patient communications regarding a denial, it's important to:

  A) Use medical jargon to explain the situation accurately

  B) Delay informing the patient until the appeals process is complete

  C) Provide clear and understandable explanations

  D) Assure the patient that denials are uncommon

5. The HIPAA Privacy Rule primarily protects:

  A) Insurance companies from fraudulent claims

  B) Patients from receiving unnecessary medical treatments

  C) The privacy of patients' health information

  D) Healthcare providers' rights to deny treatment

6. An effective appeal letter should:

  A) Be as lengthy as possible to cover all bases

  B) Include only the patient's name and date of service

  C) Outline the reasons for the appeal and include relevant supporting documentation

  D) Be written in a confrontational tone to express dissatisfaction

7. The role of financial counseling in the appeals process may involve:

   A) Providing legal advice to sue the insurance company

   B) Helping patients understand their payment options and potential financial assistance

   C) Encouraging patients to ignore the denial

   D) Assisting patients in finding alternative insurance providers

8. Regular updates during the appeal process:

   A) Are unnecessary and may confuse the patient

   B) Should be avoided to prevent raising false hope

   C) Help maintain transparency and trust with the patient

   D) Can only be given if the appeal is successful

9. A "hard denial" is characterized by:

   A) An easy resolution process

   B) The potential for reversal with minimal effort

   C) Resulting in lost or written-off revenue unless successfully appealed

   D) Being exclusively related to administrative errors

10. Patient involvement in the appeals process:

A) Is discouraged to keep the process simple

B) Can include providing additional information or direct communication with the insurer

C) Should be limited to financial contributions only

D) Is legally prohibited

Answers:

1. B) Lack of pre-authorization for a procedure

2. C) A temporary denial that may be reversed upon submission of additional information

3. C) Gathering supporting documentation and writing a concise appeal letter

4. C) Provide clear and understandable explanations

5. C) The privacy of patients' health information

6. C) Outline the reasons for the appeal and include relevant supporting documentation

7. B) Helping patients understand their payment options and potential financial assistance

8. C) Help maintain transparency and trust with the patient

9. C) Resulting in lost or written-off revenue unless successfully appealed

10. B) Can include providing additional information or direct communication with the insurer

These questions and answers are designed to enhance your comprehension of navigating insurance claim denials and appeals, emphasizing the importance of clear communication, thorough preparation, and patient support throughout the process.

Chapter 9: Medical Billing Software

9.1 Choosing the Right Software

Selecting the right medical billing software is a pivotal decision for healthcare providers, impacting the efficiency of billing operations, accuracy of claims, and overall financial health of the practice. The right software can streamline billing processes, reduce errors, and improve claim approval rates, while also enhancing patient satisfaction through transparent billing practices. Here's a guide to choosing the right medical billing software for your healthcare practice.

Key Features to Look For

1. **Comprehensive Functionality:** Look for software that supports the entire billing cycle, from patient registration and appointment scheduling to coding, claim submission, payment processing, and reporting.

2. **Ease of Use:** The interface should be intuitive and user-friendly, minimizing the learning curve for your staff and enabling efficient operation.

3. **Integration Capabilities:** Ideally, the software should integrate seamlessly with your existing Electronic Health Records (EHR) system and other practice management tools, facilitating a unified workflow.

4. **Compliance and Security:** Ensure the software complies with healthcare regulations, including HIPAA, and offers robust security features to protect patient data.

5. **Claim Scrubbing:** Advanced billing software often includes claim scrubbing features, which automatically check claims for errors and inconsistencies before submission, reducing denials and delays.

6. **Reporting and Analytics:** Look for software that provides detailed financial reporting and analytics tools, helping you monitor the financial performance of your practice and identify areas for improvement.

7. **Customization:** The ability to customize the software to fit the specific needs of your practice, including specialty-specific billing requirements, can be highly beneficial.

8. **Scalability:** Choose software that can grow with your practice, accommodating an increasing volume of patients and expanding service offerings without significant upgrades or system changes.

9. **Support and Training:** Consider the level of customer support and training provided by the software vendor. Reliable support and comprehensive training are crucial for smooth implementation and ongoing operation.

Considerations Before Making a Decision

- **Budget:** Evaluate the cost of the software against your practice's budget, considering both upfront costs and ongoing fees. Also, assess the potential return on investment through improved billing efficiency and reduced claim denials.

- **Demo and Trial:** Request a demonstration or a trial period to evaluate the software's functionality and ensure it meets your practice's needs.

- **User Reviews and References:** Research user reviews and ask for references from other healthcare providers who have implemented the software. Their insights can provide valuable information about the software's performance and reliability.

- **Vendor Reputation:** Choose a vendor with a strong reputation in the healthcare industry, known for quality software solutions and excellent customer service.

Conclusion

Selecting the right medical billing software requires careful consideration of your practice's specific needs, budget, and long-term goals. By prioritizing key features such as ease of use, compliance, integration capabilities, and robust support, healthcare providers can make an informed decision that enhances billing efficiency, ensures regulatory compliance, and ultimately contributes to the financial success of the practice.

9.2 Utilizing Billing Software Features

Once the right medical billing software has been selected, fully utilizing its features can significantly enhance the efficiency and accuracy of billing processes, improve the financial health of the practice, and elevate patient satisfaction. Effective use of billing software goes beyond basic functionality; it involves leveraging all available tools to streamline operations, reduce errors, and facilitate better communication. Here are key strategies for maximizing the benefits of your medical billing software.

Comprehensive Training

- **Initial and Ongoing Training:** Ensure all staff members are thoroughly trained on the software at the outset. Schedule regular update sessions to keep the team informed about new features or changes.

- **Role-Specific Training:** Tailor training sessions to the specific roles of your staff. For example, front-desk personnel may need extensive knowledge of scheduling and patient registration features, while billing specialists focus on claim submission and tracking.

Automating Routine Tasks

- **Automated Patient Verification:** Use software features that automatically verify patient insurance eligibility and benefits before appointments, reducing the chances of claim denials for coverage issues.

- **Claim Scrubbing:** Activate and rely on the software's claim scrubbing features to catch common coding errors, incomplete information, or discrepancies before submission, enhancing the claim acceptance rate.

Integration with EHR Systems

- **Seamless Data Flow:** Ensure the billing software is fully integrated with your EHR system, allowing for a seamless flow of patient information and minimizing the need for duplicate data entry.

- **Real-Time Access to Patient Data:** Utilize the integration to access comprehensive patient data in real-time, supporting accurate coding and billing based on detailed medical records.

Enhancing Patient Communication

- **Patient Portals:** Encourage patients to use the software's patient portal for accessing billing information, making payments, and communicating with your practice. This can improve transparency and patient satisfaction.

- **Automated Billing Updates:** Set up automated notifications or statements to keep patients informed about their billing status, payment due dates, and any outstanding balances.

Exploiting Reporting and Analytics

- **Financial Performance Analysis:** Regularly review the software's financial reports and analytics to gain insights into the practice's revenue cycle, identify trends in claim denials, and assess the effectiveness of billing practices.

- **Custom Reports:** Use the software's capabilities to generate custom reports tailored to your practice's needs, facilitating data-driven decision-making.

Maintaining Compliance

- **Regular Updates:** Keep the software updated to ensure compliance with the latest billing regulations and coding standards. Software updates often include necessary adjustments for regulatory changes.

- **Data Security:** Utilize the software's security features, such as encryption and access controls, to protect patient information and comply with HIPAA and other privacy regulations.

Leveraging Support Services

- **Vendor Support:** Take advantage of the software vendor's support services for troubleshooting, advice on best practices, or assistance with implementing new features.

- **User Community:** Engage with the user community, if available, to share experiences, tips, and strategies for maximizing the software's utility.

Conclusion

Effectively utilizing medical billing software requires a proactive approach, involving comprehensive training, automation of routine tasks, seamless integration with EHR systems, and active engagement with patients through digital tools. By exploiting the full range of features offered by billing software, healthcare practices can achieve greater efficiency, accuracy, and patient satisfaction, contributing to improved financial performance and compliance with healthcare regulations.

9.3 Troubleshooting Common Software Issues

Even the most reliable medical billing software can encounter issues that disrupt the billing process, affect productivity, and potentially impact revenue. Being prepared to identify and troubleshoot common software problems is essential for minimizing downtime and maintaining a smooth billing operation. This section outlines strategies for addressing frequent challenges encountered with medical billing software.

Data Synchronization Problems

Symptoms: Discrepancies between patient records in the EHR and billing software, or delayed updates to patient accounts.

Solutions:

- **Check Network Connectivity:** Ensure all systems are connected to the network and can communicate with the central server or cloud service.

- **Verify Integration Settings:** Review the integration settings between the EHR and billing software to ensure they are correctly configured.

- **Manual Sync:** If automatic synchronization fails, look for an option to manually initiate a sync process within the software.

Incorrect Billing Codes and Denials

Symptoms: High rates of claim denials or rejections due to coding errors.

Solutions:

- **Use Built-in Code Verification Tools:** Activate and use any claim scrubbing or code verification features to catch errors before submission.

- **Update Code Libraries:** Ensure that your software's coding libraries (ICD, CPT, HCPCS) are up to date with the latest revisions.

- **Training:** Provide additional training for staff on proper coding practices and software utilization.

Software Performance Issues

Symptoms: Slow software response times, crashes, or other performance-related problems.

Solutions:

- **Check System Requirements:** Ensure your hardware meets the software's minimum system requirements. Upgrading hardware might be necessary for optimal performance.

- **Software Updates:** Regularly update the billing software to the latest version to fix known bugs and improve stability.

- **Clear Cache/Temporary Files:** Over time, temporary files can accumulate and slow down software performance. Look for an option to clear these files within the software or consult the vendor for guidance.

Access and Permission Errors

Symptoms: Users unable to access certain features or data within the software.

Solutions:

- **Review User Roles and Permissions:** Check the assigned roles and permissions for affected users to ensure they have the correct access levels.

- **Reset Passwords:** If access issues are related to login problems, resetting the user's password can often resolve the issue.

- **Contact Support:** For complex permission issues, contacting the software vendor's support team can provide a resolution.

Integration Failures

Symptoms: Poor communication or data transfer errors between the billing software and other systems (EHR, payment processors, etc.).

Solutions:

- **Re-establish Connections:** Attempt to disconnect and then reconnect the integration links between systems, following the vendor's instructions.

- **Check for Updates:** Ensure all integrated systems are updated to compatible versions.

- **Vendor Support:** If integration issues persist, seek assistance from the software vendors involved to diagnose and resolve interoperability problems.

Conclusion

Troubleshooting common software issues is a vital skill for ensuring the continuity and efficiency of medical billing processes. By understanding the typical problems and their solutions, billing staff can quickly address challenges, reducing the impact on the practice's operations. Regular software updates, ongoing staff training, and open lines of communication with software vendors are key strategies for preventing and resolving issues, ultimately supporting the practice's financial health and patient satisfaction.

9.4 Exercise: 10 MCQs with Answers at the End

Test your knowledge on medical billing software, focusing on choosing the right software, utilizing its features, and troubleshooting common issues. This exercise is designed to reinforce your understanding of managing medical billing processes effectively using software solutions.

Questions:

1. What feature is essential for medical billing software to ensure compliance with healthcare regulations?

   A) Social media integration

   B) HIPAA compliance and security features

   C) Video game access for patient entertainment

   D) Built-in email client

2. Automated claim scrubbing helps to:

   A) Increase the number of denials

   B) Catch common coding errors before submission

   C) Slow down the billing process

   D) Automatically pay denied claims

3. Integration with Electronic Health Records (EHR) systems is important because it:

   A) Reduces the need for clinical care

   B) Minimizes manual data entry and potential errors

   C) Makes medical billing software more expensive

D) Is required by all insurance companies

4. Regular updates to medical billing software are crucial for:

A) Increasing the size of the software on the hard drive

B) Ensuring the software remains compatible with older computers

C) Keeping the software aligned with the latest billing regulations and coding standards

D) Making the user interface more complicated

5. A common issue with medical billing software that can lead to claim denials is:

A) Excessive speed of the software

B) Incorrect billing codes and denials due to coding errors

C) Too many features available for users

D) Integration with too many EHR systems

6. When choosing medical billing software, scalability is important because it:

A) Ensures the software can handle a larger volume of patients as the practice grows

B) Guarantees the software will work on all types of computers

C) Means the software can be used for non-medical billing purposes

D) Reduces the overall cost of the software over time

7. Data synchronization problems in medical billing software could lead to:

A) Faster claim processing times

B) Discrepancies between patient records in the EHR and billing software

C) An increase in the software's speed and efficiency

D) Lower costs for healthcare providers

8. Which strategy is effective for troubleshooting software performance issues?

A) Ignoring updates to avoid changes

B) Clearing cache/temporary files to improve performance

C) Using the software on older computers only

D) Decreasing the number of patients to reduce software use

9. Effective patient communication regarding billing software features could include:

A) Discouraging patients from asking questions

B) Providing access to and training on using patient portals

C) Sending all communications via postal mail only

D) Limiting information about billing to reduce patient anxiety

10. What is a benefit of utilizing reporting and analytics features in medical billing software?

   A) Ignoring data to focus on intuition

   B) Generating detailed financial reports to monitor practice performance

   C) Reducing the amount of data available for decision-making

   D) Increasing the complexity of the billing process

Answers:

1. B) HIPAA compliance and security features

2. B) Catch common coding errors before submission

3. B) Minimizes manual data entry and potential errors

4. C) Keeping the software aligned with the latest billing regulations and coding standards

5. B) Incorrect billing codes and denials due to coding errors

6. A) Ensures the software can handle a larger volume of patients as the practice grows

7. B) Discrepancies between patient records in the EHR and billing software

8. B) Clearing cache/temporary files to improve performance

9. B) Providing access to and training on using patient portals

10. B) Generating detailed financial reports to monitor practice performance

These questions and answers aim to enhance your comprehension of the complexities involved in selecting, utilizing, and troubleshooting medical billing software, ensuring you're equipped to handle the challenges of modern medical billing processes.

Chapter 10: Patient Billing and Collections

10.1 Generating Patient Bills

Generating patient bills is a crucial step in the healthcare revenue cycle, directly impacting the financial health of healthcare providers and the satisfaction of patients. This process involves creating accurate, comprehensible bills for services rendered, ensuring that patients understand their financial responsibilities and healthcare providers receive timely payments. Here's an overview of the key aspects involved in generating patient bills.

Understanding the Billing Process

The process begins once the medical services have been provided, and the claim has been processed by the insurance company. The balance, after insurance contributions (if any), is what generally constitutes the patient's bill. This process includes:

- **Review of Services Provided:** Ensuring all services rendered are accurately documented and coded.

- **Insurance Claim Processing:** Submitting claims to the insurance company and receiving payment or denial. The insurance payment, patient co-pays, deductibles, and any non-covered services are considered when generating the bill.

- **Itemization of Services:** Creating a detailed list of services provided, including dates of service, the procedures performed, associated costs, and payments received from insurance.

Key Components of an Effective Patient Bill

1. **Clarity and Detail:** Bills should clearly itemize each service provided, along with the associated cost, in a way that's understandable to patients without a medical background.

2. **Transparency:** Include detailed information about insurance payments, adjustments, deductibles, co-pays, and any outstanding balance owed by the patient.

3. **Payment Instructions:** Provide clear instructions on how to make a payment, including acceptable payment methods, due dates, and late payment policies.

4. **Contact Information:** Offer direct contact details for the billing department to address questions or concerns about the bill.

Strategies for Generating Patient-Friendly Bills

- **Simplify Language:** Use layman's terms to describe medical services and avoid medical jargon that might confuse the patient.

- **Visual Aids:** Incorporate charts or graphs to visually break down costs, payments, and balances.

- **Billing Summaries:** Alongside detailed itemizations, include a summary section that highlights the total charges, payments made by insurance, and the amount due by the patient.

- **Digital Access:** Offer electronic billing options through patient portals, allowing patients to view, manage, and pay their bills online.

Legal and Ethical Considerations

- **Compliance:** Ensure billing practices comply with healthcare regulations, including the Health Insurance Portability and Accountability Act (HIPAA) for patient privacy.

- **Accuracy:** Bills must accurately reflect the services provided and the corresponding charges. Inaccurate billing can lead to disputes, loss of patient trust, and potential legal issues.

- **Financial Assistance Policies:** Clearly communicate any available financial assistance programs or payment plans for patients experiencing financial hardship.

Conclusion

Generating patient bills is more than just a routine administrative task; it's an important part of the patient care continuum. Effective patient billing requires a balance between accuracy, clarity, and compassion. By adopting patient-friendly billing practices, healthcare providers can enhance patient satisfaction, improve the transparency of healthcare costs, and streamline the collections process, ultimately contributing to a positive healthcare experience for patients and a stable financial environment for providers.

10.2 Collection Strategies

Effective collection strategies are vital for maintaining the financial stability of healthcare practices. These strategies balance the need to collect payments while maintaining a positive relationship with patients. Implementing compassionate, efficient, and compliant collection practices can significantly reduce outstanding balances and improve cash flow. Here's how healthcare providers can optimize their collection efforts.

Pre-Service Financial Policies

- **Clear Communication of Financial Policies:** Ensure patients are aware of your financial policies, including payment expectations, at the time of service registration or appointment scheduling.

- **Verification of Insurance and Eligibility:** Confirm insurance coverage and eligibility before services are rendered to understand the coverage limits and patient responsibility.

- **Pre-Service Payment:** Implement a policy for collecting co-pays, deductibles, or estimated patient responsibilities upfront, reducing the amount to be collected post-service.

Post-Service Collection Efforts

- **Timely Billing:** Send bills promptly after services are rendered and insurance payments have been applied, ensuring that patient responsibilities are communicated clearly and early.

- **Payment Plans:** Offer flexible payment plans for patients who cannot pay their balance in full. Structured plans can help manage patient debt while ensuring steady cash flow for the practice.

- **Follow-Up and Reminders:** Utilize follow-up calls, emails, or text messages as reminders for outstanding balances. Regular communication keeps the bill at the forefront of the patient's mind without seeming aggressive.

Utilizing Technology

- **Automated Billing Systems:** Use medical billing software to automate invoicing, payment reminders, and tracking of patient accounts, improving efficiency and reducing manual errors.

- **Online Patient Portals:** Encourage the use of online portals where patients can view their bills, make payments, and set up payment plans conveniently.

- **Electronic Payment Options:** Offer various electronic payment methods, including credit/debit cards, online payments, and mobile payment platforms, making it easier for patients to fulfill their financial obligations.

Patient Communication and Education

- **Financial Counseling:** Provide financial counseling services to help patients understand their bills, insurance benefits, and available financial assistance or payment options.

- **Transparency:** Be transparent about costs and patient responsibilities from the outset. Clear and open communication can prevent confusion and disputes down the line.

Dealing with Delinquent Accounts

- **Compassionate Approach:** Approach delinquent accounts with empathy, understanding that patients may be facing financial hardships. Exploring all options and working with the patient can often lead to a resolution.

- **Third-Party Collection Agencies:** As a last resort, consider partnering with a reputable collection agency that specializes in healthcare and adheres to ethical collection practices. Ensure they comply with the Fair Debt Collection Practices Act (FDCPA) and other relevant regulations.

Regulatory Compliance

- **Adhere to Regulations:** Ensure all collection practices comply with federal and state regulations, including the FDCPA, HIPAA, and state-specific consumer protection laws.

- **Training Staff:** Regularly train staff on ethical and legal collection practices, emphasizing respectful and compassionate patient interactions.

Conclusion

Optimizing collection strategies involves a combination of upfront communication, leveraging technology for efficiency, compassionate patient engagement, and adherence to regulatory standards. By implementing these practices, healthcare providers can improve collections, maintain positive patient relationships, and ensure the financial health of their practice.

10.3 Handling Patient Inquiries

Effectively handling patient inquiries about billing and collections is essential for maintaining patient trust and satisfaction. Patients often have questions regarding their bills, insurance coverage, payment options, or the specifics of the services they received. Providing clear, concise, and compassionate responses not only helps resolve patient concerns but also reinforces a positive relationship between healthcare providers and patients. Here's a guide to managing patient billing inquiries effectively.

Establishing a Responsive System

- **Dedicated Billing Support:** Establish a dedicated team or individual responsible for handling billing inquiries. This ensures that patients have a direct line to someone knowledgeable about billing processes.

- **Multiple Channels for Inquiries:** Offer various channels for patients to make inquiries, including phone, email, online patient portals, and in-person visits. Ensure these channels are monitored regularly for timely responses.

Training Staff

- **Comprehensive Training:** Provide comprehensive training for staff handling billing inquiries, covering the billing process, common patient questions, and the practice's policies on payments and financial assistance.

- **Customer Service Skills:** Emphasize the importance of customer service skills, including active listening, empathy, and clear communication. Staff should be prepared to handle inquiries with patience and understanding.

Effective Communication Strategies

- **Clarity and Transparency:** Use clear and understandable language when explaining billing matters. Avoid medical and billing jargon that might confuse patients.

- **Personalized Responses:** Tailor responses to the individual patient's inquiry, providing specific information related to their bill or account status.

- **Follow-Up:** If an issue cannot be resolved immediately, ensure timely follow-up communication with the patient. Keep them informed about the status of their inquiry.

Utilizing Technology

- **Patient Portals:** Encourage the use of online patient portals where patients can view detailed billings, payment histories, and insurance information. Portals can also be a convenient channel for asking questions and receiving responses.

- **Automated Information:** Implement automated systems for common inquiries, such as balance checks or payment confirmations, allowing patients to access information quickly without waiting for a staff response.

Documenting Inquiries

- **Record Keeping:** Keep detailed records of all patient inquiries and responses. Documentation can help in resolving future disputes, improving billing processes, and identifying areas for service improvement.

- **Feedback Loop:** Use patient inquiries as feedback to identify common billing issues or areas of confusion. This insight can guide improvements in the billing process and patient communication materials.

Handling Sensitive Conversations

- **Financial Hardship:** Be prepared to handle conversations with patients experiencing financial hardship. Offer information on payment plans, financial assistance, and other resources to help them manage their bills.

- **Disputes and Complaints:** Approach disputes and complaints with a problem-solving mindset. Listen to the patient's concerns, investigate the issue, and work collaboratively towards a resolution.

Conclusion

Handling patient billing inquiries with efficiency, empathy, and transparency is crucial for fostering trust and ensuring patient satisfaction. By establishing responsive systems, training staff, leveraging technology, and maintaining open lines of communication, healthcare providers can effectively address patient concerns, mitigate confusion, and support their financial well-being.

10.4 Exercise: 10 MCQs with Answers at the End

Test your understanding of patient billing and collections, including generating patient bills, collection strategies, and handling patient inquiries. This exercise aims to reinforce key practices that ensure financial health for healthcare providers and maintain patient satisfaction.

Questions:

1. What is a key element in generating patient-friendly bills?

   A) Using complex medical jargon for accuracy

   B) Delaying the bill as long as possible to increase payment amounts

   C) Clarity and detail in itemization

   D) Limiting payment options to direct bank transfers only

2. Effective collection strategies should include:

   A) Ignoring patient financial hardships

   B) Flexible payment plans for patients who cannot pay in full

   C) Avoiding discussions about outstanding balances

   D) Sending bills without detailed explanations

3. When establishing a responsive system for handling billing inquiries, it's important to:

   A) Offer only one way for patients to contact your office

   B) Train staff extensively in all aspects of patient care, not just billing

   C) Provide multiple channels for patients to make inquiries

D) Discourage patients from asking questions to reduce workload

4. An effective strategy for dealing with delinquent accounts is:

A) Immediate referral to a collection agency

B) Compassionate communication and offering payment solutions

C) Ignoring the account in hopes it resolves itself

D) Increasing the total amount owed as a penalty

5. The use of patient portals in billing can:

A) Confuse patients further without offering any real benefits

B) Enhance patient satisfaction by offering transparency and convenience

C) Reduce the efficiency of the billing process

D) Only benefit the healthcare provider, not the patient

6. Automated claim scrubbing features are designed to:

A) Slow down the billing process by adding extra steps

B) Increase the number of claim denials for educational purposes

C) Catch common coding errors before submission to reduce denials

D) Automatically pay any denied claims without review

7. A dedicated billing support team helps by:

   A) Decreasing the overall efficiency of the billing process

   B) Increasing the complexity of patient inquiries

   C) Ensuring knowledgeable staff are available to answer patient questions

   D) Making it harder for patients to receive personalized responses

8. Regular updates to medical billing software ensure that:

   A) The software becomes incompatible with other systems over time

   B) Billing practices remain aligned with the latest regulations and standards

   C) Staff become confused by constant changes

   D) The software requires frequent reinstallation

9. Pre-service financial policies are effective for:

   A) Discouraging patients from seeking care

   B) Clearly communicating payment expectations upfront

   C) Reducing the quality of patient care

   D) Creating barriers between patients and providers

10. Training staff in customer service skills for handling billing inquiries is crucial because:

   A) It prevents patients from understanding their bills

   B) It helps manage patient frustrations and concerns with empathy and clarity

   C) Technical knowledge is irrelevant in billing inquiries

   D) It encourages staff to avoid patient interactions

Answers:

1. C) Clarity and detail in itemization

2. B) Flexible payment plans for patients who cannot pay in full

3. C) Provide multiple channels for patients to make inquiries

4. B) Compassionate communication and offering payment solutions

5. B) Enhance patient satisfaction by offering transparency and convenience

6. C) Catch common coding errors before submission to reduce denials

7. C) Ensuring knowledgeable staff are available to answer patient questions

8. B) Billing practices remain aligned with the latest regulations and standards

9. B) Clearly communicating payment expectations upfront

10. B) It helps manage patient frustrations and concerns with empathy and clarity

These questions and answers are designed to deepen your understanding of the intricacies involved in patient billing and collections, highlighting the importance of clarity, compassion, and compliance in these processes.

Chapter 11: Auditing and Quality Assurance

11.1 Principles of Medical Billing Audits

Medical billing audits are essential components of quality assurance in healthcare practices. They serve to verify the accuracy of billing operations, ensure compliance with coding standards and regulations, and identify areas for improvement in the revenue cycle management process. Understanding the principles of medical billing audits can help practices maintain financial integrity, minimize compliance risks, and enhance patient satisfaction.

Purpose of Medical Billing Audits

- **Compliance Verification:** Audits check for adherence to federal, state, and payer-specific billing and coding regulations, including HIPAA and other healthcare laws.

- **Accuracy Improvement:** They identify inaccuracies in coding, documentation, and billing processes that could lead to claim denials or compliance issues.

- **Revenue Optimization:** Audits can uncover undercoding or missed billing opportunities, ensuring that the practice receives appropriate reimbursement for the services provided.

- **Educational Opportunity:** Audit findings can serve as a basis for training and educating staff on proper coding and billing practices.

Types of Medical Billing Audits

1. **Internal Audits:** Conducted by the practice's own staff or hired consultants, internal audits provide a proactive approach to identifying and correcting issues before they result in external scrutiny.

2. **External Audits:** Performed by outside entities, such as Medicare contractors, insurance companies, or regulatory agencies, external audits are typically more formal and can have significant implications.

Key Components of an Effective Audit Process

- **Selection of Claims:** Audits should randomly select a representative sample of claims that reflects the diversity of services provided, payer mix, and coding complexities.

- **Review Process:** The review should encompass a comprehensive examination of documentation, coding, billing data, and compliance with payer policies.

- **Benchmarking:** Comparing audit findings against industry benchmarks or standards helps to gauge the practice's performance and identify areas for improvement.

- **Reporting:** Detailed reports should outline the findings, including specific examples of errors or discrepancies, and recommend corrective actions.

- **Action Plan:** Develop and implement an action plan based on audit findings to address identified issues, improve processes, and prevent future errors.

Best Practices for Conducting Medical Billing Audits

- **Regular Schedule:** Establish a regular schedule for audits, whether quarterly, semi-annually, or annually, to consistently monitor and improve billing practices.

- **Confidentiality and Objectivity:** Ensure that audits are conducted in a confidential manner and that the auditors maintain objectivity, without biases towards any staff members or departments.

- **Follow-up and Monitoring:** After implementing corrective actions, monitor their effectiveness over time and consider follow-up audits to ensure sustained improvement.

- **Staff Involvement and Education:** Involve staff in the audit process and use audit findings as educational tools to foster a culture of continuous improvement and compliance.

Conclusion

Medical billing audits are vital for ensuring the accuracy and compliance of billing operations in healthcare practices. By adhering to the principles of effective auditing, practices can identify and rectify issues, optimize revenue, and maintain high standards of compliance and patient care. Regular, systematic audits, combined with targeted education and improvement initiatives, form the cornerstone of a robust quality assurance program in medical billing.

11.2 Conducting an Effective Audit

Conducting an effective audit in the realm of medical billing is a meticulous process that requires a clear understanding of billing practices, regulatory compliance, and the specific goals of the audit. Whether the audit is internal or external, its effectiveness hinges on thorough preparation, execution, and follow-up. Here are the key steps involved in conducting an effective audit in medical billing.

Preparation Phase

1. **Define the Scope and Objectives:** Clearly outline what the audit aims to achieve, whether it's to verify compliance with specific regulations, assess the accuracy of coding, or evaluate the effectiveness of billing processes.

2. **Develop an Audit Plan:** Create a detailed plan that includes the selection criteria for claims, timelines, necessary resources, and the personnel involved. The plan should align with the audit's objectives and ensure comprehensive coverage of billing activities.

3. **Select a Representative Sample:** Choose a random sample of claims that represents the variety of services provided, different payers, and the range of coding complexities encountered in the practice. The sample size should be sufficient to provide reliable insights into overall billing practices.

Execution Phase

1. **Review Documentation:** Examine patient records, billing documents, and claims submissions for the selected sample. Verify that the documentation supports the services billed and that coding is accurate and compliant with current standards.

2. **Identify Errors and Issues:** Look for common issues such as incomplete documentation, incorrect coding, lack of necessary authorizations, and non-compliance with payer policies. Note any patterns or trends in the errors identified.

3. **Assess Compliance:** Evaluate the practice's adherence to relevant regulations and guidelines, including HIPAA, False Claims Act, and payer-specific rules.

Reporting and Follow-Up Phase

1. **Compile Findings:** Summarize the audit findings, highlighting key issues, error rates, and areas for improvement. Include specific examples and references to coding guidelines or regulations where applicable.

2. **Develop Recommendations:** Based on the audit findings, propose actionable recommendations for correcting identified issues, enhancing billing processes, and preventing future errors. Recommendations may include staff training, process changes, or the implementation of new controls.

3. **Present the Audit Report:** Share the report with key stakeholders, including management, billing staff, and healthcare providers. Ensure the presentation is clear, concise, and focuses on constructive solutions.

4. **Create an Action Plan:** Collaborate with the relevant teams to develop an action plan that addresses the audit's recommendations. Assign responsibilities, set deadlines, and establish metrics for measuring improvement.

5. **Monitor Progress and Implement Changes:** Regularly monitor the implementation of the action plan, making adjustments as necessary. Consider conducting follow-up audits to assess the effectiveness of the changes made.

Best Practices for Conducting Audits

- **Maintain Objectivity:** Ensure that the audit is conducted impartially and objectively, without preconceived notions influencing the findings.

- **Ensure Confidentiality:** Protect the confidentiality of patient information and sensitive practice data throughout the audit process.

- **Promote Transparency:** Communicate openly with staff about the purpose and process of the audit, fostering a culture of transparency and continuous improvement.

- **Leverage Technology:** Utilize medical billing software and auditing tools to streamline the audit process and enhance the accuracy of the review.

Conclusion

Conducting an effective audit in medical billing is a critical exercise for ensuring compliance, accuracy, and efficiency. By following a structured approach from preparation through to follow-up, healthcare practices can identify areas for improvement, mitigate risks, and ultimately enhance their financial and operational performance.

11.3 Quality Assurance in Billing

Quality assurance (QA) in medical billing is a systematic process aimed at ensuring the accuracy, reliability, and compliance of billing practices. This ongoing effort helps healthcare providers to minimize errors, optimize revenue, and maintain a positive reputation among patients and payers alike. Implementing a robust QA program involves several key components and strategies designed to uphold high standards in billing operations.

Core Components of Quality Assurance in Billing

1. **Standard Operating Procedures (SOPs):** Develop and document clear SOPs for all billing processes, including patient registration, coding, claim submission, and handling denials and appeals. SOPs ensure consistency and compliance across the billing department.

2. **Regular Training and Education:** Provide continuous training for billing staff on the latest coding standards, billing software updates, and changes in healthcare regulations. This keeps the team informed and reduces the likelihood of errors.

3. **Auditing and Monitoring:** Conduct regular audits of billing practices, as described in earlier sections, to identify and correct inaccuracies. Continuous monitoring allows for the early detection of issues before they escalate.

4. **Feedback Loop:** Establish a mechanism for receiving and incorporating feedback from billing staff, healthcare providers, and patients. This feedback can offer valuable insights into areas needing improvement.

5. **Technology Utilization:** Leverage advanced billing software and tools that offer features like automated claim scrubbing, error alerts, and analytics. These technologies can significantly enhance the accuracy and efficiency of billing operations.

Strategies for Ensuring Quality in Billing

- **Error Tracking and Analysis:** Implement a system for tracking billing errors, categorizing them by type and cause. Regular analysis of this data helps identify patterns and areas for targeted improvement.

- **Performance Metrics:** Define key performance indicators (KPIs) for the billing process, such as the rate of claim denials, average days in accounts receivable (A/R), and the percentage of clean claims. Monitor these metrics closely to assess the effectiveness of your QA efforts.

- **Collaboration with Clinical Staff:** Foster strong communication and collaboration between billing staff and clinical providers. This ensures that documentation accurately reflects the services provided, supporting correct coding and billing.

- **Patient Communication:** Enhance patient communication regarding billing matters. Clear, transparent billing statements and accessible customer service can reduce patient complaints and improve satisfaction.

- **Corrective Action Plans:** When issues are identified, develop and implement corrective action plans promptly. This may involve retraining staff, revising SOPs, or making changes to billing software settings.

Benefits of Quality Assurance in Billing

- **Reduced Billing Errors:** A strong QA program leads to fewer billing and coding errors, reducing claim denials and rejections.

- **Improved Financial Performance:** Accurate and efficient billing processes optimize revenue collection and shorten the revenue cycle.

- **Regulatory Compliance:** Adherence to billing regulations and guidelines minimizes the risk of audits, penalties, and reputational damage.

- **Enhanced Patient Satisfaction:** Transparent, accurate billing practices improve patient trust and satisfaction, contributing to patient retention and positive reviews.

Conclusion

Quality assurance in medical billing is not a one-time effort but a continuous process of evaluation and improvement. By committing to QA, healthcare practices can ensure their billing operations are accurate, compliant, and efficient, ultimately supporting their financial health and fostering trust among patients and payers.

11.4 Exercise: 10 MCQs with Answers at the End

Test your understanding of auditing and quality assurance in medical billing with these multiple-choice questions. This exercise is designed to reinforce the principles, processes, and benefits of implementing effective audit and QA practices in healthcare billing.

Questions:

1. What is the primary goal of medical billing audits?

   A) To increase the workload of billing staff

   B) To verify compliance and improve accuracy

   C) To intimidate the billing staff

D) To reduce the number of patients

2. Regular training and education for billing staff are important for:

A) Keeping the staff occupied

B) Meeting the minimum legal requirements

C) Staying updated on coding standards and regulations

D) Increasing staff turnover

3. A key component of quality assurance in billing is:

A) Avoiding the use of technology

B) Manual processing of all claims

C) Regular auditing and monitoring

D) Decreasing patient communication

4. Effective quality assurance strategies include:

A) Ignoring feedback from clinical staff

B) Error tracking and analysis

C) Limiting access to billing records

D) Encouraging billing errors as learning opportunities

5. The use of advanced billing software and tools can:

    A) Complicate the billing process unnecessarily

    B) Enhance the accuracy and efficiency of billing operations

    C) Discourage staff from learning basic coding

    D) Increase the risk of compliance violations

6. Collaborating with clinical staff in the billing process helps to:

    A) Undermine the authority of the billing department

    B) Ensure documentation accurately reflects services provided

    C) Create confusion and delays in billing

    D) Reduce the need for accurate coding

7. The establishment of Standard Operating Procedures (SOPs) in billing is meant to:

    A) Confuse new staff members

    B) Increase variability in billing practices

    C) Ensure consistency and compliance

    D) Make the audit process more difficult

8. A feedback loop in the billing process is important for:

    A) Ignoring constructive criticism

    B) Identifying areas needing improvement

    C) Maintaining outdated practices

D) Reducing staff participation

9. One benefit of quality assurance in medical billing is:

A) Increased claim denials

B) Reduced billing errors

C) Slower revenue cycle

D) Higher patient dissatisfaction

10. Performance metrics in billing might include all except:

A) Rate of claim denials

B) Average days in accounts receivable (A/R)

C) Number of staff coffee breaks

D) Percentage of clean claims

Answers:

1. B) To verify compliance and improve accuracy

2. C) Staying updated on coding standards and regulations

3. C) Regular auditing and monitoring

4. B) Error tracking and analysis

5. B) Enhance the accuracy and efficiency of billing operations

6. B) Ensure documentation accurately reflects services provided

7. C) Ensure consistency and compliance

8. B) Identifying areas needing improvement

9. B) Reduced billing errors

10. C) Number of staff coffee breaks

These questions and answers aim to enhance your comprehension of the importance and implementation of auditing and quality assurance in the medical billing process, emphasizing continuous improvement and adherence to best practices.

Chapter 12: Revenue Cycle Management

12.1 Overview of Revenue Cycle

Revenue Cycle Management (RCM) is a critical aspect of healthcare administration that encompasses all the financial processes involved in managing the administrative and clinical functions associated with claims processing, payment, and revenue generation. The revenue cycle starts from the moment a patient makes an appointment and continues through the delivery of services, billing, and final payment. Understanding the revenue cycle's components and how they interconnect can help healthcare organizations optimize their processes, improve patient satisfaction, and maximize financial performance.

Key Components of the Revenue Cycle

1. **Patient Registration and Pre-authorization:** The cycle begins when a patient schedules an appointment. Collecting accurate patient information and verifying insurance eligibility and benefits are crucial steps to prevent delays and denials.

2. **Charge Capture and Coding:** Services provided to the patient are documented and translated into billable charges using appropriate coding systems, such as ICD-10, CPT, and HCPCS

codes. Accurate coding is essential for billing and reimbursement.

3. **Claim Submission:** Prepared claims are submitted to insurance companies or payers for reimbursement. Claims must adhere to payer-specific guidelines to avoid rejections or denials.

4. **Payment Posting:** Payments received from payers are posted to the patient accounts. This step involves reconciling the amounts paid against the claims submitted.

5. **Patient Billing:** After insurance payments are applied, any remaining balance is billed to the patient. Clear and accurate bills are essential for timely patient payments.

6. **Denial Management:** Denied claims are reviewed, corrected, and resubmitted as necessary. Effective denial management processes can significantly impact revenue recovery.

7. **Accounts Receivable Follow-up:** This involves monitoring outstanding balances, both with payers and patients, and taking action to resolve delayed payments or underpayments.

Challenges in Revenue Cycle Management

- **Complexity of Payer Contracts:** Navigating the various terms and conditions of payer contracts can be challenging and requires detailed attention.

- **Regulatory Compliance:** Staying compliant with healthcare regulations and coding standards is an ongoing challenge that requires continuous education and vigilance.

- **Denials and Rejections:** Managing denials and rejections efficiently to minimize revenue loss and improve cash flow is a critical aspect of RCM.

- **Patient Financial Responsibility:** With the rise in high-deductible health plans, collecting payments from patients has become increasingly complex and crucial for maintaining revenue.

Strategies for Optimizing Revenue Cycle Management

- **Leverage Technology:** Implement advanced RCM software solutions that automate processes, reduce manual errors, and provide analytics for better decision-making.

- **Improve Patient Engagement:** Enhance patient communication and education regarding their financial responsibilities and payment options.

- **Staff Training:** Regularly train staff on the latest billing practices, coding updates, and regulatory requirements.

- **Outsource When Necessary:** Consider outsourcing challenging aspects of RCM, such as coding or collections, to specialized companies that can offer expertise and efficiency.

- **Continuous Process Improvement:** Regularly review and refine RCM processes to identify bottlenecks, eliminate inefficiencies, and adopt best practices.

Conclusion

Effective revenue cycle management is vital for the financial health of healthcare organizations. By understanding and optimizing each component of the revenue cycle, healthcare providers can ensure accurate billing, timely reimbursements, and ultimately, sustained financial viability and the ability to provide quality patient care.

12.2 Improving Cash Flow

Improving cash flow within the context of Revenue Cycle Management (RCM) is crucial for the financial health and operational sustainability of healthcare organizations. Efficient cash flow management ensures that practices have the necessary funds to cover operational costs, invest in technology, and improve patient care services. Here are strategies to enhance cash flow in healthcare settings.

Streamline Front-End Processes

- **Accurate Patient Registration:** Ensure patient information is accurate and complete at the time of registration to prevent billing errors and claim denials.

- **Insurance Verification:** Verify insurance eligibility and benefits for each patient before service delivery to ascertain coverage and patient financial responsibility.

- **Pre-Authorization:** Obtain necessary pre-authorizations for procedures and services to ensure they will be covered by the patient's insurance plan.

Optimize Charge Capture and Coding

- **Comprehensive Documentation:** Encourage thorough documentation of services provided to capture all chargeable items accurately.

- **Regular Coding Updates:** Stay updated with the latest coding guidelines and ensure coding practices are compliant with current standards to maximize claim reimbursement.

- **Utilize Charge Capture Technology:** Implement automated charge capture systems to reduce missed charges and improve billing accuracy.

Efficient Claim Management

- **Timely Claim Submission:** Submit claims as soon as possible after service delivery to accelerate reimbursements.

- **Claim Scrubbing:** Use claim scrubbing tools to identify and correct errors before submission, reducing the likelihood of denials and delays.

- **Denial Management:** Implement a robust process for quickly addressing and resubmitting denied claims to recover revenue promptly.

Enhance Accounts Receivable (A/R) Management

- **A/R Follow-Up:** Actively follow up on outstanding claims with payers and overdue patient balances to ensure timely payment.

- **Clear Aging Buckets:** Focus on clearing older A/R first, particularly those over 90 days, as they are harder to collect over time.

- **Payment Plan Options:** Offer flexible payment plans to patients who cannot pay their balances in full, improving cash collections while maintaining patient satisfaction.

Leverage Technology and Analytics

- **RCM Software Solutions:** Use RCM software that provides real-time analytics and reporting tools to monitor key financial metrics and identify areas for improvement.

- **Automated Alerts and Reminders:** Set up automated systems for patient payment reminders and follow-ups on pending insurance claims to reduce the time to payment.

Patient Payment Policies

- **Upfront Payment Policies:** Clearly communicate payment policies to patients, including the collection of copays and deductibles at the time of service.

- **Transparent Billing:** Provide clear and understandable bills to patients, reducing confusion and disputes that can delay payments.

Outsourcing When Necessary

- **Specialized RCM Services:** Consider outsourcing challenging aspects of RCM, such as billing and collections, to specialized firms that can offer expertise, efficiency, and improved results.

Regular Training and Education

- **Staff Training:** Continuously train staff on best practices in billing, coding, and collections to ensure they are equipped to manage the revenue cycle effectively.

Conclusion

Improving cash flow in healthcare requires a comprehensive approach that spans the entire revenue cycle. By focusing on front-end processes, optimizing billing and coding practices, managing claims efficiently, and enhancing patient payment policies, healthcare organizations can significantly improve their cash flow, ensuring financial stability and the ability to deliver high-quality care.

12.3 Key Performance Indicators

In Revenue Cycle Management (RCM), Key Performance Indicators (KPIs) are crucial metrics that help healthcare organizations measure the efficiency and effectiveness of their billing and collections processes. Tracking these indicators provides insights into operational performance, identifies areas for improvement, and aids in strategic decision-making. Here are some of the essential KPIs for assessing the health of a healthcare organization's revenue cycle.

Days in Accounts Receivable (A/R)

- **Definition:** The average number of days it takes for an organization to collect payments due.

- **Importance:** Lower A/R days indicate faster collection times, improving cash flow. High A/R days may signal issues with claim submissions or collections processes.

Clean Claim Rate

- **Definition:** The percentage of claims paid on the first submission without requiring correction or additional information.

- **Importance:** A high clean claim rate reduces the time and resources spent on reworking claims, leading to quicker reimbursements.

Claim Denial Rate

- **Definition:** The percentage of claims denied by payers.

- **Importance:** A low denial rate suggests effective billing practices and accurate coding. High denial rates necessitate a review of the billing process to identify and rectify common denial reasons.

Net Collection Rate

- **Definition:** The percentage of total potential reimbursement collected from all sources.

- **Importance:** This KPI measures the effectiveness of the collections process. Rates close to 100% indicate that the organization is successfully collecting the revenue it is entitled to.

Cost to Collect

- **Definition:** The total cost associated with collecting payments from payers and patients.

- **Importance:** Lower costs to collect indicate more efficient billing and collections operations, maximizing the revenue retained by the organization.

Time to Payment

- **Definition:** The average time from the date of service or claim submission to the date payment is received.

- **Importance:** Shorter payment times enhance cash flow, enabling the organization to reinvest in operations and patient care more quickly.

Patient Responsibility Rate

- **Definition:** The percentage of revenue coming directly from patients, as opposed to insurance payers.

- **Importance:** With the rise of high-deductible health plans, monitoring this rate helps organizations understand the changing landscape of patient payments and adjust their collection strategies accordingly.

Implementing KPI Monitoring

- **Regular Reporting:** Generate regular reports on these KPIs to monitor trends over time.

- **Benchmarking:** Compare KPIs against industry benchmarks or historical performance to gauge success and identify areas for improvement.

- **Actionable Insights:** Use KPI data to make informed decisions about process changes, staff training needs, or technology investments.

Conclusion

Key Performance Indicators are vital tools in managing the revenue cycle efficiently. By systematically tracking and analyzing these metrics, healthcare organizations can pinpoint operational strengths and weaknesses, optimize billing and collection processes, and ultimately achieve financial stability while continuing to provide high-quality patient care.

12.4 Exercise: 10 MCQs with Answers at the End

Test your knowledge on Revenue Cycle Management (RCM) with these multiple-choice questions. This exercise is designed to reinforce your understanding of the overview of the revenue cycle, strategies to improve cash flow, key performance indicators, and overall best practices in RCM.

Questions:

1. What is the first step in the Revenue Cycle Management process?

   A) Claim submission

   B) Patient registration and pre-authorization

   C) Payment posting

   D) Denial management

2. The purpose of charge capture and coding in RCM is to:

   A) Decrease the overall revenue

   B) Ensure patient data privacy

   C) Translate services into billable charges

   D) Increase patient wait times

3. A clean claim rate refers to:

A) The cleanliness of the physical billing documents

B) Claims paid on the first submission without needing additional information

C) The percentage of claims denied by payers

D) The speed at which claims are processed by software

4. Improving cash flow in RCM can be achieved by:

A) Delaying claim submissions

B) Ignoring denied claims

C) Offering flexible payment plans to patients

D) Increasing the cost of services

5. Days in Accounts Receivable (A/R) measures:

A) The average cost of submitting a claim

B) How quickly a practice pays its bills

C) The average number of days it takes to collect payments due

D) The number of days an account remains delinquent

6. A high net collection rate indicates:

A) Ineffective collection processes

B) The practice is collecting a high percentage of the revenue it is owed

C) The practice is overcharging patients

D) A high rate of claim denials

7. The cost to collect is important because:

A) It measures patient satisfaction with billing processes

B) Lower costs indicate more efficient billing and collection operations

C) It directly influences the number of services provided

D) Higher costs always indicate better quality of care

8. Effective denial management in RCM involves:

A) Accepting all denials as final

B) Quickly addressing and resubmitting denied claims

C) Increasing the time between denial receipt and resubmission

D) Eliminating the process of appeal for denied claims

9. Patient responsibility rate has become an important KPI due to:

A) Decreases in insurance coverage for many services

B) The rise of high-deductible health plans

C) Patients preferring to pay out of pocket

D) Legislation requiring upfront payment for all healthcare services

10. Regular training and education for staff are crucial in RCM to:

A) Reduce the efficiency of the billing process

B) Ensure compliance with changing regulations and coding standards

C) Limit the use of advanced billing software

D) Decrease staff morale and job satisfaction

Answers:

1. B) Patient registration and pre-authorization

2. C) Translate services into billable charges

3. B) Claims paid on the first submission without needing additional information

4. C) Offering flexible payment plans to patients

5. C) The average number of days it takes to collect payments due

6. B) The practice is collecting a high percentage of the revenue it is owed

7. B) Lower costs indicate more efficient billing and collection operations

8. B) Quickly addressing and resubmitting denied claims

9. B) The rise of high-deductible health plans

10. B) Ensure compliance with changing regulations and coding standards

These questions and answers aim to deepen your understanding of Revenue Cycle Management, emphasizing the importance of each step in the process, strategies for optimization, and the significance of monitoring key performance indicators for successful RCM.

Chapter 13: Dealing with Special Populations

13.1 Billing for Pediatric Patients

Billing for pediatric patients involves unique challenges and considerations that healthcare providers must navigate carefully. Pediatric billing encompasses services for patients from birth through adolescence, requiring an understanding of specific coding nuances, preventive care guidelines, and family dynamics. Here's a guide to effectively manage billing for pediatric populations.

Understanding Pediatric Billing Nuances

- **Preventive Care and Immunizations:** Pediatric care emphasizes preventive services, which include well-child visits, immunizations, and developmental screenings. These services often have specific coding guidelines and may be covered differently by insurance plans.

- **Age-Specific Codes:** Certain procedures and services in pediatrics are billed based on the patient's age, necessitating careful attention to coding to ensure accurate reimbursement.

- **Family Accounts:** Billing for pediatric patients often involves managing family accounts where multiple family members receive care within the same practice, requiring a system that can accurately track individual and family deductibles and co-payments.

Best Practices for Pediatric Billing

1. **Stay Updated on Preventive Care Guidelines:** Regularly review and update billing practices based on the latest preventive care guidelines and immunization schedules to ensure compliance with coding and billing for these services.

2. **Verify Insurance Coverage:** Because pediatric coverage can vary widely among insurance plans, especially for preventive care and immunizations, verify coverage details and benefits for each patient at the time of service.

3. **Utilize Age-Specific Codes Accurately:** Ensure that billing staff are trained to use age-specific codes correctly and are aware of the age ranges that impact billing and coding for pediatric services.

4. **Coordinate with Families:** Communicate clearly with parents or guardians about their insurance benefits, out-of-pocket responsibilities, and any applicable family deductibles. Providing education on insurance coverage can help prevent billing surprises and disputes.

5. **Manage Family Accounts Efficiently:** Implement billing software that supports family accounts management, allowing for the accurate tracking of deductibles and co-payments across family members.

6. **Document Thoroughly:** Maintain detailed documentation of all services provided, including preventive care and counseling, to support claims and minimize denials.

7. **Handle Vaccines Carefully:** Vaccines can be a significant expense in pediatric care. Understand the billing nuances for vaccines, including the use of vaccine administration codes and the Vaccine For Children (VFC) program where applicable.

8. **Engage in Advocacy:** Stay informed about changes in healthcare policy affecting pediatric care and engage in advocacy efforts to support favorable coverage for pediatric services.

Challenges in Pediatric Billing

- **Complexity of Coverage:** Navigating the complexities of insurance coverage for pediatric services, especially with variations in coverage for preventive services and vaccines.

- **Coordination of Benefits:** Managing cases where multiple insurance policies may cover the pediatric patient, requiring coordination of benefits.

- **Billing for Developmental and Behavioral Services:** Coding and billing for developmental and behavioral assessments and treatments can be complex, with specific documentation requirements.

Conclusion

Billing for pediatric patients requires a specialized approach that accounts for the unique aspects of pediatric care, insurance coverage, and family dynamics. By adhering to best practices in pediatric billing, healthcare providers can ensure accurate reimbursement while supporting the health and well-being of their youngest patients. Navigating these challenges effectively not only enhances revenue cycle management but also contributes to the delivery of high-quality pediatric care.

13.2 Addressing Elderly Patient Needs

Billing for elderly patients, often covered under Medicare or supplemental insurance plans, presents unique challenges and considerations. This demographic typically requires management of chronic conditions, multiple medications, and potentially frequent healthcare services. Understanding the nuances of billing for elderly patients is crucial for healthcare providers to ensure accurate reimbursement and compliance, while also addressing the specific needs and concerns of this patient population.

Understanding Medicare and Supplemental Insurance

- **Medicare Coverage:** Familiarize yourself with Medicare Parts A, B, C, and D, including what services each part covers and the associated billing guidelines. Medicare often serves as the primary insurance for elderly patients.

- **Supplemental Insurance:** Many elderly patients have supplemental insurance to cover costs not fully reimbursed by Medicare. Understanding how to coordinate benefits and bill secondary insurance is essential.

- **Medicare Advantage Plans (Part C):** Be aware of the specifics of Medicare Advantage plans, which may have different billing requirements and networks compared to traditional Medicare.

Best Practices for Billing Elderly Patients

1. **Verify Coverage and Benefits:** Prior to services, verify each patient's Medicare and any supplemental insurance coverage, including deductibles, copayments, and specific coverage limitations or requirements.

2. **Pre-Authorization and Referral Requirements:** Check for any pre-authorization or referral requirements, especially for patients enrolled in Medicare Advantage plans, to ensure services will be covered.

3. **Accurate Coding:** Use appropriate diagnosis codes that accurately reflect the patient's condition, particularly for chronic conditions common in elderly patients. Ensure coding compliance with Medicare guidelines.

4. **Medication Management Billing:** For elderly patients on multiple medications, services such as Medication Therapy Management (MTM) may be billable under certain conditions. Be familiar with the billing criteria for these services.

5. **Chronic Care Management (CCM) Services:** Medicare provides reimbursement for CCM services for patients with multiple chronic conditions. Understand the requirements for billing these services, including the need for patient consent and detailed documentation.

6. **Utilize Preventive Service Benefits:** Medicare covers various preventive services, such as annual wellness visits and screenings, without copayments. Educating patients about these benefits can improve care while ensuring reimbursement for provided services.

Addressing Elderly Patient Concerns

- **Clear Communication:** Provide clear explanations of covered services, out-of-pocket costs, and the billing process to reduce confusion and anxiety for elderly patients.

- **Patient Advocacy:** Assist patients in understanding their Medicare benefits and supplemental insurance, and advocate on their behalf with insurance providers as needed.

- **Billing Inquiries:** Establish a responsive system for handling billing inquiries specific to elderly patients, ensuring staff are knowledgeable about Medicare and supplemental insurance.

Challenges in Elderly Patient Billing

- **Navigating Medicare Rules:** Keeping up-to-date with frequently changing Medicare rules and regulations can be challenging.

- **Coordinating Benefits:** Managing the coordination of benefits between Medicare and supplemental insurance requires meticulous attention to detail.

- **Addressing Social Determinants of Health:** Elderly patients may face issues such as fixed incomes or lack of transportation, which can impact their ability to receive care. Being sensitive to these factors and exploring supportive services is important.

Conclusion

Billing for elderly patients requires a comprehensive understanding of Medicare, supplemental insurance plans, and the unique healthcare needs of this population. By implementing best practices tailored to elderly patient billing, healthcare providers can ensure compliance, optimize reimbursement, and support the health and well-being of their elderly patients, fostering trust and satisfaction.

13.3 Managing Billing for Disabled Patients

Billing for disabled patients encompasses a broad range of challenges and considerations, reflective of the diverse needs of this patient population. Disabilities can vary widely in nature and severity, including physical, intellectual, and developmental disabilities, each requiring specific accommodations and understanding from healthcare providers. Effective billing practices for disabled patients not only ensure compliance and reimbursement but also promote accessibility, equity, and compassionate care.

Key Considerations in Billing for Disabled Patients

- **Understanding Coverage:** Disabled patients may have coverage through various sources, including Medicaid, Medicare (if they qualify for Social Security Disability Insurance), private insurance, or disability-specific programs. Familiarity with each of these programs' billing guidelines is crucial.

- **Accessibility and Communication:** Ensure that billing processes and communications are accessible to all patients, including those with visual, hearing, or cognitive impairments. This may involve providing billing statements in large print, Braille, or easy-to-understand language.

- **Coordinated Care Needs:** Disabled patients often require services from multiple healthcare providers and specialists. Coordinating care and billing across providers is essential to avoid duplicate charges and ensure comprehensive coverage.

Strategies for Effective Billing

1. **Verify Insurance Coverage and Benefits:** Conduct thorough verification of insurance benefits for each disabled patient, taking into account the possibility of multiple coverage sources. Determine the primary payer and understand the coordination of benefits rules.

2. **Pre-Authorization and Documentation:** Obtain necessary pre-authorizations for treatments and ensure all services are documented accurately and comprehensively. Proper documentation supports the medical necessity of services, a critical factor in securing reimbursement.

3. **Customized Billing Statements:** Customize billing statements to meet the specific needs of disabled patients, ensuring they are understandable and accessible. Consider the patient's method of communication and adapt accordingly.

4. **Flexible Payment Options:** Offer flexible payment options and plans to accommodate the financial situations of disabled patients, who may be on a fixed income due to their disability.

5. **Staff Training:** Train billing staff on the nuances of billing for disabled patients, including sensitivity training and familiarity with the various insurance programs and accommodations required.

6. **Utilize Patient Advocates:** Employ patient advocates or case managers to assist disabled patients in navigating their healthcare, including understanding their coverage, bills, and the appeals process for denied claims.

Challenges and Solutions

- **Complexity of Coverage:** Disabled patients' coverage can be complex. Solution: Establish a dedicated team or point of contact within the billing department specializing in this area.

- **Billing for Long-term and Comprehensive Services:** Disabled patients may require long-term, comprehensive services. Solution: Ensure accurate coding and leverage chronic care management and other relevant billing codes.

- **Communication Barriers:** Effective communication with disabled patients about billing may require special accommodations. Solution: Implement a variety of communication methods tailored to the needs of disabled patients.

Conclusion

Managing billing for disabled patients requires a multifaceted approach that respects the diversity and specific needs of this patient population. By ensuring accessibility, understanding coverage intricacies, and providing compassionate and tailored billing support, healthcare providers can enhance the billing experience for disabled patients. This not only facilitates compliance and reimbursement but also reinforces a commitment to inclusive, equitable healthcare.

13.4 Exercise: 10 MCQs with Answers at the End

Test your knowledge on dealing with special populations in medical billing, covering pediatric, elderly, and disabled patients. This exercise aims to reinforce your understanding of the unique billing considerations and best practices for these diverse patient groups.

Questions:

1. Which insurance is typically the primary coverage for most elderly patients?

   A) Private insurance

   B) Medicaid

C) Medicare

D) Employer-sponsored insurance

2. Preventive care and immunizations in pediatric billing are important because:

A) They are always fully covered by insurance.

B) They require special age-specific codes.

C) Parents request them the most.

D) They are optional services.

3. When billing for disabled patients, what is a crucial factor to ensure reimbursement?

A) Increasing the billing cycle time

B) Documenting the medical necessity of services

C) Limiting communication methods

D) Using a one-size-fits-all approach to billing statements

4. Flexible payment options are particularly important for which patient group, due to potential fixed incomes?

A) Pediatric patients

B) Elderly patients

C) Disabled patients

D) All of the above

5. Coordination of benefits is a significant consideration when billing for:

   A) Elderly patients only

   B) Disabled patients only

   C) Both elderly and disabled patients

   D) Pediatric patients only

6. Accessible billing communications for disabled patients may require:

   A) Standard print materials only

   B) Braille or large print options

   C) Email communications exclusively

   D) Phone calls only

7. The primary purpose of Medicaid for pediatric patients is to:

   A) Cover all healthcare costs without co-payments

   B) Provide a supplement to Medicare

   C) Serve as the primary insurance coverage for low-income families

   D) Replace private insurance

8. Customized billing statements for patients with disabilities are essential for:

   A) Making the billing process more complex

   B) Ensuring compliance with federal regulations

   C) Enhancing the aesthetic appeal of billing documents

   D) Facilitating understanding and accessibility

9. In pediatric billing, managing family accounts requires attention to:

   A) Only the oldest child's medical expenses

   B) Individual and family deductibles and co-payments

   C) Ignoring insurance verification processes

   D) Billing all services under the parent's name only

10. A key challenge in billing for elderly patients involves:

   A) Navigating the complexities of Medicare and supplemental insurance

   B) The absence of preventive care services

   C) Decreased need for medical services

   D) Simplified billing codes and processes

Answers:

1. C) Medicare

2. B) They require special age-specific codes.

3. B) Documenting the medical necessity of services

4. C) Disabled patients

5. C) Both elderly and disabled patients

6. B) Braille or large print options

7. C) Serve as the primary insurance coverage for low-income families

8. D) Facilitating understanding and accessibility

9. B) Individual and family deductibles and co-payments

10. A) Navigating the complexities of Medicare and supplemental insurance

These questions and answers aim to deepen your understanding of the specialized considerations required when billing for pediatric, elderly, and disabled patients, highlighting the importance of tailored approaches to meet the diverse needs of these patient groups effectively.

Chapter 14: Telemedicine Billing

14.1 Introduction to Telemedicine

Telemedicine, the remote delivery of healthcare services using telecommunications technology, has seen a significant rise in adoption among healthcare providers and patients. It offers an innovative way to provide clinical services when in-person visits are not necessary or possible. This shift towards virtual care has necessitated a parallel evolution in billing practices to accommodate the nuances of telemedicine services. Understanding the basics of telemedicine and its billing implications is crucial for healthcare providers looking to integrate this modality into their practice efficiently and compliantly.

What is Telemedicine?

Telemedicine involves the use of electronic communications and software to provide clinical services to patients without an in-person visit. Services may include consultations, examinations, monitoring, and even certain therapies, all conducted via video conferencing, secure messaging, or other digital platforms.

Benefits of Telemedicine

- **Accessibility:** Makes healthcare more accessible, especially for patients in remote areas or those with mobility issues.

- **Convenience:** Reduces the need for travel, saving time for both patients and providers.

- **Efficiency:** Can lead to more efficient use of healthcare resources, reducing the burden on physical healthcare facilities.

- **Patient Satisfaction:** Often results in high levels of patient satisfaction due to convenience and accessibility.

Billing for Telemedicine Services

Billing for telemedicine services presents unique challenges, including understanding payer policies, coding correctly for telehealth services, and navigating state laws and regulations. Here's an overview of key considerations:

- **Payer Policies:** Telemedicine coverage varies by payer, including Medicare, Medicaid, and private insurance companies. Providers must verify whether a payer covers telemedicine services and understand the specific requirements for coverage.

- **Coding and Reimbursement:** Proper coding is essential for telemedicine billing. This includes using the correct CPT/HCPCS codes, modifiers (e.g., GT or 95 for synchronous telehealth services), and place of service (POS) codes to indicate that the service was delivered via telemedicine.

- **State Regulations:** Telemedicine regulations can vary significantly by state, affecting licensure, consent, reimbursement, and other aspects of telehealth practice. Providers must ensure compliance with the regulations in the state where the patient is located at the time of service.

- **Documentation:** As with in-person visits, thorough documentation of telemedicine services is critical for billing and compliance. Providers should document the technology used, the duration of the visit, and the nature of the services provided.

Challenges in Telemedicine Billing

- **Interstate Licensure:** Providing services across state lines may require providers to hold licenses in the patient's state, complicating billing and compliance.

- **Technology Requirements:** Ensuring privacy and security in telehealth platforms is essential for compliance with HIPAA and other regulations, impacting the choice of technology and platforms for telemedicine services.

- **Patient Awareness:** Educating patients about the availability, benefits, and costs associated with telemedicine can affect its adoption and the billing process.

Conclusion

Telemedicine represents a significant advancement in healthcare delivery, offering benefits to both patients and providers. However, navigating the billing and regulatory landscape requires a clear understanding of payer policies, state regulations, and appropriate coding practices. As telemedicine continues to evolve, staying informed about these aspects will be crucial for healthcare providers to successfully integrate telemedicine into their practice and ensure proper reimbursement for these services.

14.2 Coding for Telehealth Services

With the expansion of telehealth services, understanding the appropriate coding practices becomes crucial for healthcare providers to ensure accurate billing and reimbursement. Telehealth coding involves specific codes, modifiers, and guidelines that indicate a service was delivered remotely. Here's an overview of key coding principles for telehealth services to navigate this complex landscape effectively.

Key Coding Components for Telehealth

1. **CPT/HCPCS Codes:** The use of standard CPT (Current Procedural Terminology) and HCPCS (Healthcare Common Procedure Coding System) codes applies to telehealth services, similar to in-person services. The selection of codes will depend

on the nature of the service provided (e.g., consultation, evaluation and management, mental health services).

2. **Modifiers:** Modifiers are used in conjunction with CPT/HCPCS codes to further describe the circumstances of the service. For telehealth, common modifiers include:

- **95 Modifier:** Indicates a synchronous telemedicine service rendered via a real-time interactive audio and video telecommunications system.

- **GT Modifier (via interactive audio and video telecommunications systems):** Historically used for Medicare claims to signify telehealth services, though CMS now generally prefers the 95 modifier.

- **GQ Modifier:** Used for services delivered via asynchronous telecommunications system in specific circumstances.

3. **Place of Service (POS) Codes:** The POS code indicates where the service was performed. For telehealth, the POS code often used is:

- **POS 02 (Telehealth):** Indicates that the service was provided remotely as part of a telehealth encounter.

- **Changes During COVID-19:** During the public health emergency, providers were allowed to bill telehealth services using the POS code that would have been used if the service had been provided in person, along with a 95 modifier to indicate telehealth delivery.

Billing Considerations and Best Practices

- **Payer-Specific Guidelines:** Be aware that payer guidelines for telehealth coding and reimbursement can vary. Always verify current policies with each payer to ensure compliance and accurate billing.

- **Documentation:** Maintain comprehensive documentation for telehealth services, including the duration of the visit, the technology used, and consent for telehealth (as required by some payers or states).

- **State Regulations and Licensure:** Understand the impact of state regulations on telehealth services, including licensure requirements for providing services to out-of-state patients.

- **Telehealth during COVID-19:** The COVID-19 pandemic led to temporary expansions in telehealth coverage and flexibility in billing practices. Stay updated on the latest guidance from CMS and other payers as these policies may evolve post-pandemic.

Emerging Trends and Future Directions

- **Expansion of Telehealth Services:** As telehealth continues to grow, new codes and guidelines are likely to emerge, addressing the evolving nature of remote healthcare delivery.

- **Permanent Policy Changes:** The temporary expansions in telehealth coverage due to COVID-19 may lead to permanent changes in telehealth policy, coding, and reimbursement practices.

Conclusion

Coding for telehealth services requires a detailed understanding of the appropriate use of CPT/HCPCS codes, modifiers, and POS codes that accurately reflect telehealth encounters. By staying informed of payer-specific guidelines and regulatory changes, especially in the evolving landscape post-COVID-19, healthcare providers can ensure proper billing and maximize reimbursement for telehealth services.

14.3 Reimbursement for Telemedicine

Reimbursement for telemedicine services has evolved significantly, especially with the increased adoption of telehealth during the COVID-19 pandemic. Understanding the landscape of telemedicine reimbursement is crucial for healthcare providers to navigate billing practices effectively and ensure financial viability for their telehealth programs. This overview addresses key aspects of telemedicine reimbursement, including payer policies, regulatory considerations, and strategies to maximize reimbursement.

Payer Policies on Telemedicine Reimbursement

- **Medicare:** Traditionally, Medicare reimbursed telehealth services under specific conditions, such as services provided to patients in rural areas. However, emergency measures during the COVID-19 pandemic expanded coverage to include a broader range of services and locations. Providers should stay informed about permanent changes post-pandemic.

- **Medicaid:** State Medicaid programs have their own policies regarding telehealth reimbursement, with most states expanding coverage for telehealth services. The flexibility and scope of coverage vary by state.

- **Private Insurers:** Many private insurance companies have expanded telehealth coverage in response to COVID-19, with some making these changes permanent. Policies vary widely among insurers, so providers must verify coverage and reimbursement rates for telehealth services with each insurer.

Regulatory Considerations

- **Licensure:** Providers must be licensed in the state where the patient is located at the time of service, which can affect reimbursement eligibility for telehealth services across state lines.

- **Consent:** Some payers and states require documented patient consent for telehealth services, impacting reimbursement if not properly obtained and recorded.

- **Interstate Compacts and Emergency Regulations:** The Interstate Medical Licensure Compact and temporary emergency regulations in response to COVID-19 have facilitated cross-state telehealth services. Providers should be aware of these regulations' impact on reimbursement.

Strategies to Maximize Telemedicine Reimbursement

1. **Verify Coverage and Pre-Authorization:** Before providing telehealth services, verify that the patient's insurance plan covers the services and if pre-authorization is required to ensure reimbursement.

2. **Accurate Coding and Documentation:** Use the correct telehealth-specific codes, modifiers, and place of service codes. Ensure documentation meets payer requirements for telehealth services, including the technology used and the duration of the visit.

3. **Stay Updated on Payer Policies:** Regularly review and stay informed about changes in telehealth reimbursement policies for Medicare, Medicaid, and private insurers, as these can evolve rapidly.

4. **Educate Staff:** Ensure billing and coding staff are trained on the latest telehealth billing practices and payer policies to avoid errors that could lead to claim denials.

5. **Negotiate with Private Payers:** For practices with significant telehealth services, consider negotiating telehealth reimbursement rates with private payers to ensure adequate compensation for services provided.

Emerging Trends and Future Directions

The future of telemedicine reimbursement is likely to see further evolution as healthcare delivery continues to integrate telehealth into standard practice. Advocacy for more comprehensive telehealth coverage, permanent policy changes post-pandemic, and the development of new billing codes to reflect telehealth services are areas to watch.

Conclusion

Reimbursement for telemedicine services requires a comprehensive understanding of current payer policies, regulatory requirements, and effective billing practices. By adopting strategies to navigate these complexities, healthcare providers can secure appropriate reimbursement for telehealth services, supporting the sustainability of telemedicine programs and expanding access to care for patients.

14.4 Exercise: 10 MCQs with Answers at the End

Test your knowledge on telemedicine billing, covering introduction to telemedicine, coding for telehealth services, and reimbursement strategies. This exercise is designed to reinforce key aspects of telemedicine billing practices.

Questions:

1. What modifier is commonly used to indicate a telemedicine service delivered via a real-time interactive audio and video telecommunications system?

   A) GT

   B) 95

   C) GQ

   D) QQ

2. Medicare's coverage of telehealth services was traditionally limited to patients in:

   A) Urban areas only

   B) Any location

   C) Rural areas with limited healthcare access

   D) State capitals

3. For telehealth services, what Place of Service (POS) code is often used?

   A) 02

   B) 11

   C) 22

   D) 50

4. During the COVID-19 pandemic, Medicare temporarily allowed telehealth services to be billed:

A) Only for COVID-19 related treatments

B) Using the same POS codes as if the service had been provided in person

C) Without any reimbursement

D) Exclusively for mental health services

5. State Medicaid programs typically:

A) Do not cover telehealth services

B) Have uniform telehealth coverage across all states

C) Have their own policies regarding telehealth reimbursement

D) Only cover telehealth for pediatric patients

6. Accurate documentation for telehealth services MUST include:

A) The patient's preference for telehealth over in-person visits

B) The technology used and the duration of the visit

C) The patient's location at the time of billing, not service

D) A transcript of the entire telehealth conversation

7. Pre-authorization for telehealth services is:

   A) Never required by any payer

   B) Required by all payers without exception

   C) Dependent on the payer's policies

   D) Only necessary for international patients

8. A key challenge in telemedicine billing is:

   A) Simplified coding options for telehealth services

   B) Navigating varying payer policies and state regulations

   C) Higher reimbursement rates for telehealth than in-person visits

   D) Universal coverage for all telehealth services by private insurers

9. Private insurers have responded to the increased use of telehealth by:

   A) Decreasing coverage for all digital health services

   B) Expanding telehealth coverage, with some making changes permanent

   C) Covering telehealth only for select specialties

   D) Requiring higher copayments for telehealth than in-person services

10. To maximize reimbursement for telemedicine services, providers should:

   A) Use general codes for all telehealth visits to simplify billing

   B) Assume all telehealth services are covered equally across all payers

   C) Verify coverage and pre-authorization requirements with each payer

   D) Limit telehealth services to only those patients who request them

Answers:

1. B) 95

2. C) Rural areas with limited healthcare access

3. A) 02

4. B) Using the same POS codes as if the service had been provided in person

5. C) Have their own policies regarding telehealth reimbursement

6. B) The technology used and the duration of the visit

7. C) Dependent on the payer's policies

8. B) Navigating varying payer policies and state regulations

9. B) Expanding telehealth coverage, with some making changes permanent

10. C) Verify coverage and pre-authorization requirements with each payer

These questions and answers aim to deepen your understanding of the complexities involved in telemedicine billing, emphasizing the importance of accurate coding, understanding payer policies, and ensuring compliance with documentation and regulatory requirements.

Chapter 15: Specialty Medical Billing

15.1 Billing for Surgery and Anesthesia

Billing for surgery and anesthesia presents unique challenges and requires specialized knowledge due to the complexity of procedures, the variety of codes, and specific payer policies. Understanding the nuances of billing in these specialties is crucial for accurate reimbursement and compliance with healthcare regulations.

Surgical Billing Considerations

- **Global Surgical Package:** Most surgical procedures are billed under a global package concept, which includes all necessary services normally furnished by a surgeon before, during, and after a procedure. Understanding what is included in the global package is essential to avoid unbundling or incorrect billing.

- **Procedure Codes (CPT):** Accurate Current Procedural Terminology (CPT) coding is critical. This includes selecting the right code for the surgical procedure performed and understanding any modifiers that may apply to describe the surgery's complexity, multiple procedures, or when only a portion of the standard procedure is performed.

- **Pre-Authorization:** Many surgical procedures require pre-authorization from the insurance provider to ensure coverage. Failing to obtain pre-authorization can result in denied claims.

Anesthesia Billing Considerations

- **Time Reporting:** Anesthesia billing is unique because it often involves billing based on the duration the patient is under anesthesia. Accurately reporting start and stop times is crucial for correct billing.

- **Base Units and Time Units:** Anesthesia billing combines base units (reflecting the complexity of the procedure) with time units (the duration of anesthesia) and any applicable modifiers. Understanding how to calculate and report these units is essential for accurate reimbursement.

- **Modifiers:** Specific modifiers for anesthesia billing indicate circumstances such as whether the anesthesia was personally performed, medically directed, or medically supervised. Correct use of these modifiers is necessary for proper payment.

Strategies for Effective Billing in Surgery and Anesthesia

1. **Stay Updated on Coding Guidelines:** Regularly review updates to CPT codes and anesthesia billing guidelines, as these can change annually.

2. **Comprehensive Documentation:** Ensure detailed documentation of the surgical procedure, including any

unexpected complications or additional procedures, and detailed anesthesia records to support billing claims.

3. **Verify Coverage and Benefits:** Before scheduling surgery, verify the patient's insurance coverage, benefits, and any pre-authorization requirements to anticipate potential billing issues.

4. **Use of Billing Software:** Leverage specialized medical billing software that can handle the complexities of surgery and anesthesia billing, including the calculation of anesthesia time units and the application of global surgical packages.

5. **Regular Audits:** Conduct regular billing audits to identify and correct common errors, such as undercoding, overcoding, or incorrect use of modifiers, which can lead to claim denials or compliance issues.

Challenges in Billing for Surgery and Anesthesia

- **Complex Payer Policies:** Navigating the various and often complex payer policies specific to surgery and anesthesia can be challenging.

- **Modifier Application:** Incorrect application of modifiers can lead to denied claims or reduced reimbursement.

- **Regulatory Compliance:** Ensuring compliance with healthcare regulations, including accurate reporting and documentation, is paramount to avoid penalties.

Conclusion

Billing for surgery and anesthesia requires a detailed understanding of specific coding practices, payer policies, and regulatory requirements unique to these specialties. By employing effective strategies such as staying current with coding updates, ensuring comprehensive documentation, and leveraging technology, healthcare providers can navigate the complexities of billing for these services, ensuring accurate reimbursement and maintaining compliance with healthcare regulations.

15.2 Oncology Billing Considerations

Billing for oncology services involves navigating a complex landscape of treatment modalities, coding intricacies, and payer-specific guidelines. Oncology encompasses a wide range of services, including chemotherapy, radiation therapy, hormonal therapy, and targeted therapy, each with its own billing challenges. Effective oncology billing requires an understanding of the specific considerations and best practices tailored to the oncology field.

Unique Aspects of Oncology Billing

1. **Treatment Plans:** Oncology treatments often involve comprehensive plans that span several months and include

various modalities. Understanding the entirety of a patient's treatment plan is crucial for accurate billing and reimbursement.

2. **Drug Administration Codes:** Chemotherapy and other drug therapies require precise coding for the administration of each drug. This includes specific codes for the method of administration (e.g., intravenous, oral) and the drugs themselves.

3. **Modifiers:** Given the complexity of oncology treatments, the use of modifiers is common and essential for accurate billing. Modifiers may indicate whether a service was part of a clinical trial, if multiple therapies were given on the same day, or If services were rendered outside the standard treatment plan.

4. **Payer Policies:** Oncology billing is heavily influenced by individual payer policies, which can vary widely. These policies may dictate coverage for specific drugs, treatments, and procedures, often based on the diagnosis and stage of cancer.

Strategies for Effective Oncology Billing

1. **Thorough Verification of Benefits:** Before beginning treatment, verify the patient's insurance benefits, focusing on coverage for oncology services, drug formularies, and any limitations or caps on coverage.

2. **Accurate Documentation:** Detailed documentation is critical, including diagnosis, treatment plans, administered drugs, dosages, and any adverse reactions. Documentation supports medical necessity and aids in dispute resolution with payers.

3. **Stay Updated on Coding Changes:** Oncology coding guidelines, including CPT, HCPCS, and ICD-10 codes, are frequently updated. Staying informed about these changes ensures compliance and maximizes reimbursement.

4. **Utilize Technology:** Employ oncology-specific billing software or modules capable of handling the complexities of oncology treatments, including regimen-based billing and the tracking of cumulative drug dosages.

5. **Engage with Payer Policies:** Develop a deep understanding of payer policies related to oncology treatments. Engaging with payers about coverage can help clarify ambiguities and prevent claim denials.

Challenges in Oncology Billing

- **Managing Drug Costs:** The high cost of oncology drugs, especially novel therapies, can pose reimbursement challenges. Billing accurately for these drugs while managing patient out-of-pocket costs requires careful planning.

- **Compliance with Regulations:** Oncology billing must adhere to strict regulations, including those related to clinical trials and off-label drug use. Non-compliance can lead to audits, penalties, and reimbursement issues.

- **Patient Financial Responsibility:** Communicating with patients about their financial responsibility, especially given the high costs associated with cancer treatment, is essential for maintaining transparency and trust.

Conclusion

Oncology billing is characterized by its complexity and the critical need for precision in every aspect of the billing process. By employing strategic approaches to documentation, coding, and payer engagement, practices can navigate the challenges inherent in oncology billing. Effective billing practices not only ensure proper reimbursement but also support the provision of high-quality care to patients navigating their cancer treatment journey.

15.3 Billing for Mental Health Services

Billing for mental health services encompasses a unique set of challenges and considerations, reflecting the distinct nature of these services compared to other medical fields. Mental health billing involves navigating specific coding nuances, understanding payer policies for behavioral health, and addressing the confidentiality concerns inherent in mental health treatment. Here's an overview of key considerations and best practices for effective billing in mental health care.

Unique Aspects of Mental Health Billing

1. **Diagnosis Codes:** Mental health services rely heavily on the accurate use of ICD-10 codes to describe psychiatric diagnoses. Correct diagnosis coding is crucial for reimbursement and requires a deep understanding of the ICD-10 classification for mental and behavioral disorders.

2. **Service Codes:** CPT codes for mental health services cover a range of services, including psychiatric evaluations, psychotherapy sessions (of varying durations), group therapy, and crisis intervention. Familiarity with these codes and their specific requirements is essential.

3. **Session Length:** Many mental health CPT codes are time-based, reflecting the duration of therapy sessions. Billing staff must accurately track and report session lengths to ensure proper reimbursement.

4. **Telehealth for Mental Health:** The rise of telehealth has been particularly significant in mental health care. Billing for telehealth services requires understanding of the specific modifiers and place of service (POS) codes that indicate a service was delivered remotely.

Strategies for Effective Mental Health Billing

1. **Verify Insurance Benefits:** Prior to treatment, verify each patient's insurance benefits, focusing on coverage for mental health services, which can vary significantly from other medical services. Determine any copayments, deductibles, and session limits.

2. **Understand Payer Policies:** Payer policies for mental health services can differ widely, including restrictions on the types of providers who can bill for services and limitations on the number of covered sessions. Familiarizing yourself with these policies for each payer is critical.

3. **Accurate Documentation:** Ensure thorough documentation of all mental health services provided, including the focus of therapy, session duration, and treatment outcomes. Documentation supports the medical necessity of services and aids in appeals for denied claims.

4. **Confidentiality and Billing:** Given the sensitive nature of mental health treatment, maintaining patient confidentiality is paramount. This includes careful handling of diagnoses and treatment details in billing communications.

Challenges in Mental Health Billing

- **Parity in Mental Health Coverage:** Despite laws requiring parity in insurance coverage for mental and physical health conditions, navigating these requirements in practice can be challenging, with disparities often existing in coverage levels and reimbursement rates.

- **Pre-Authorization Requirements:** Some payers require pre-authorization for mental health services, adding an administrative layer that can delay treatment initiation.

- **Reimbursement Rates:** Mental health services often face lower reimbursement rates compared to other medical services, impacting the financial viability of providing comprehensive mental health care.

Conclusion

Billing for mental health services requires specialized knowledge of coding, payer policies, and the unique aspects of mental health care delivery. By employing effective billing practices, providers can navigate the complexities of mental health reimbursement, ensuring that patients receive the necessary care while maintaining the financial health of their practice. Staying informed about changes in mental health billing regulations and payer policies is essential for adapting to the evolving landscape of mental health care.

15.4 Exercise: 10 MCQs with Answers at the End

Test your knowledge on specialty medical billing, covering surgery and anesthesia, oncology, and mental health services. This exercise is designed to highlight the unique billing considerations and best practices for these specialized areas of healthcare.

Questions:

1. The global surgical package typically includes services provided:

   A) Only during the surgery.

   B) Before, during, and after the surgery.

   C) Only after the surgery.

   D) Only before the surgery.

2. In anesthesia billing, the total time billed for anesthesia services is determined by:

   A) The complexity of the surgery.

   B) The duration the patient is under anesthesia.

   C) The type of anesthesia used.

   D) The surgeon's experience level.

3. Oncology billing often requires special attention to:

   A) Drug administration codes.

   B) Physical therapy codes.

   C) Durable medical equipment codes.

   D) Preventive care codes.

4. Mental health billing codes are unique because:

   A) They do not require diagnosis codes.

   B) They are often time-based, reflecting the session length.

   C) They are the same as codes for physical health services.

   D) They are only used for in-person sessions.

5. Accurate coding in surgery billing is crucial for:

   A) Decreasing the global surgical package.

   B) Increasing the length of hospital stay.

   C) Ensuring proper reimbursement.

   D) Simplifying patient discharge processes.

6. When billing for telehealth mental health services, what is essential?

A) Using the same codes as for in-person services without modifiers.

B) Applying specific telehealth modifiers to indicate remote delivery.

C) Avoiding documentation of the service.

D) Billing only for sessions longer than 60 minutes.

7. Pre-authorization is crucial in oncology billing to:

A) Confirm the patient's eligibility for surgery.

B) Ensure coverage for specific drugs and treatments.

C) Decrease the need for treatment plans.

D) Simplify the coding process.

8. One challenge in mental health billing is:

A) Higher reimbursement rates compared to other medical fields.

B) Parity in insurance coverage for mental and physical health conditions.

C) The absence of confidential information in billing documents.

D) The requirement for shorter session lengths.

9. The use of base units and time units in billing is specific to:

   A) Surgery.

   B) Anesthesia.

   C) Oncology.

   D) Mental health.

10. Documentation for mental health services billing should include:

   A) Only the type of medication prescribed.

   B) Detailed notes on the focus of therapy and session duration.

   C) Generic descriptions of therapy sessions.

   D) The physical health status of the patient only.

Answers:

1. B) Before, during, and after the surgery.

2. B) The duration the patient is under anesthesia.

3. A) Drug administration codes.

4. B) They are often time-based, reflecting the session length.

5. C) Ensuring proper reimbursement.

6. B) Applying specific telehealth modifiers to indicate remote delivery.

7. B) Ensure coverage for specific drugs and treatments.

8. B) Parity in insurance coverage for mental and physical health conditions.

9. B) Anesthesia.

10. B) Detailed notes on the focus of therapy and session duration.

These questions and answers aim to enhance your understanding of the complexities involved in specialty medical billing, emphasizing the importance of accurate coding, thorough documentation, and adherence to payer policies for successful reimbursement.

Chapter 16: Hospital Billing Practices

16.1 Inpatient vs. Outpatient Billing

Hospital billing practices vary significantly depending on whether a patient is considered inpatient or outpatient. Understanding the distinctions between these two types of billing is crucial for accurate coding, compliance, and reimbursement. This overview explores the key differences and considerations for inpatient and outpatient billing in hospital settings.

Inpatient Billing

Inpatient billing applies to patients who are formally admitted to a hospital with a physician's order for an overnight stay or longer. These cases often involve more complex and comprehensive care.

Key Aspects:

- **DRG Coding:** Inpatient services are typically billed under Diagnosis-Related Groups (DRGs), which bundle the costs of services and treatments into a single charge based on the patient's diagnosis and procedures performed.

- **Global Billing:** The global charge includes all services provided during the stay, such as room charges, meals, medications, tests, and procedures.

- **Length of Stay:** The patient's length of stay can influence the DRG assignment and, consequently, the reimbursement rate.

Outpatient Billing

Outpatient billing is for patients who receive services (such as diagnostic tests, surgeries, and treatments) in a hospital setting without being admitted for an overnight stay.

Key Aspects:

- **CPT/HCPCS Coding:** Outpatient services use Current Procedural Terminology (CPT) and Healthcare Common Procedure Coding System (HCPCS) codes to bill for each specific service or procedure performed.

- **Facility Fees:** Hospitals may charge facility fees for outpatient services to cover the use of hospital space, equipment, and staff.

- **Observation Status:** Patients in observation status are treated as outpatients, even if they stay in the hospital overnight. Billing for observation services requires careful attention to payer policies and time documentation.

Distinguishing Factors

- **Admission Status:** The defining factor between inpatient and outpatient billing is the patient's admission status, determined by a physician's order for inpatient care.

- **Type of Billing Codes:** Inpatient billing relies on DRG codes, while outpatient services are billed using CPT and HCPCS codes.

- **Reimbursement Models:** Inpatient services are reimbursed based on the DRG system, which considers the overall care and diagnosis. Outpatient services are reimbursed per service or procedure.

Billing Considerations and Challenges

- **Correct Admission Status:** Incorrectly designating a patient's admission status can lead to billing errors, claim denials, and compliance issues.

- **Observation Services:** Billing for observation services can be complex, as it straddles the line between inpatient and outpatient care. Proper documentation of the observation period and medical necessity is essential.

- **Payer Policies:** Understanding the specific policies of Medicare, Medicaid, and private insurers regarding inpatient and outpatient services is crucial for accurate billing and reimbursement.

Conclusion

Accurate inpatient and outpatient billing is foundational to hospital revenue cycle management. Hospitals must carefully determine and document a patient's admission status, use the appropriate coding system, and understand payer-specific guidelines to ensure compliance and optimize reimbursement. By addressing the unique challenges of inpatient and outpatient billing, hospitals can navigate the complexities of healthcare reimbursement effectively.

16.2 Understanding DRGs and Inpatient Coding

Diagnosis-Related Groups (DRGs) play a pivotal role in the billing process for inpatient hospital services. Introduced to standardize hospital reimbursements while encouraging cost containment and quality improvement, DRGs categorize hospital cases into groups that are expected to have similar hospital resource use. Understanding DRGs and their impact on inpatient coding and billing is essential for hospital revenue cycle management.

What are DRGs?

DRGs are a classification system used to group hospital cases based on similar clinical conditions (diagnoses) and the procedures performed during the stay. Each DRG is assigned a weight reflecting the expected costliness of patient care for that group, which determines the reimbursement rate from Medicare and other payers.

Key Components of DRG Assignment

1. **Principal Diagnosis:** The main condition treated or investigated during the hospital stay.

2. **Secondary Diagnoses:** Additional conditions that coexist at the time of admission or develop during the stay, which may affect patient care.

3. **Procedures Performed:** Surgical or other procedures performed during the hospital stay.

4. **Patient Demographics:** Age, sex, and discharge status can influence DRG assignment.

5. **Complications or Comorbidities (CCs) and Major Complications or Comorbidities (MCCs):** CCs and MCCs can significantly impact the DRG weight, reflecting the increased resources needed for patients with complex conditions.

Impact on Hospital Billing and Reimbursement

- **Standardized Payments:** DRGs standardize payments for inpatient stays, ensuring hospitals are reimbursed a fixed amount for patients with similar conditions and treatments, regardless of the actual cost incurred.

- **Efficiency and Quality Incentives:** The DRG system incentivizes hospitals to manage resources efficiently and improve the quality of care, as reimbursement is not directly tied to the length of stay or services rendered.

- **Coding Accuracy:** Precise and accurate medical coding is crucial in the DRG system. Inaccurate or incomplete coding can lead to incorrect DRG assignment, affecting reimbursement and potentially leading to audits and penalties.

Challenges in DRG Coding

- **Complexity of Cases:** Coding for inpatient stays involves capturing all aspects of a patient's care, which can be complex due to multiple diagnoses and procedures.

- **Documentation:** Comprehensive and accurate documentation by healthcare providers is essential for correct DRG assignment and to justify the medical necessity of services.

- **Upcoding and Downcoding:** Ensuring coding practices accurately reflect the care provided is critical. Upcoding (overstating the severity of a patient's condition) or downcoding (understating severity) can lead to compliance issues and financial penalties.

Strategies for Effective DRG Management

1. **Education and Training:** Continual education and training for coding professionals and healthcare providers on DRG guidelines and documentation best practices.

2. **Auditing and Monitoring:** Regular internal audits to identify coding inaccuracies and areas for improvement.

3. **Collaboration Between Departments:** Effective communication and collaboration between clinical staff and coders to ensure accurate and comprehensive documentation.

Conclusion

DRGs are a fundamental component of inpatient hospital billing, affecting how services are coded and reimbursed. By ensuring accurate documentation and coding, hospitals can navigate the DRG system effectively, optimizing reimbursement while adhering to regulatory compliance. The focus on efficiency and quality of care inherent in the DRG system underscores the importance of precise inpatient coding practices in today's healthcare environment.

16.3 Managing Hospital Claim Denials

Hospital claim denials are a significant challenge in revenue cycle management, directly impacting financial performance and cash flow. Efficiently managing and preventing claim denials requires a comprehensive understanding of common denial reasons and implementing strategies to address them. This section outlines the critical aspects of managing hospital claim denials, including identification, resolution, and prevention strategies.

Common Reasons for Hospital Claim Denials

1. **Incomplete or Incorrect Patient Information:** Errors in patient data, such as misspelled names, incorrect policy numbers, or inaccurate demographic details.

2. **Lack of Pre-Authorization or Referral:** Services provided without the necessary pre-authorization or without a proper referral, when required by the insurance plan.

3. **Coding Errors:** Incorrect, outdated, or unspecific coding, including diagnosis codes (ICD-10), procedure codes (CPT/HCPCS), and modifiers.

4. **Service Not Covered:** Services rendered are not covered under the patient's insurance plan or are deemed not medically necessary.

5. **Timely Filing Violations:** Claims submitted after the payer's deadline for claim submission.

Strategies for Managing Claim Denials

- **Denial Analysis:** Regularly analyze denial data to identify patterns and common reasons for denials. This analysis can help target improvement efforts.

- **Staff Training:** Ensure that billing and coding staff are well-trained and up-to-date on payer policies, coding standards, and regulatory requirements.

- **Effective Documentation:** Enhance clinical documentation practices to ensure that medical records accurately and comprehensively reflect the care provided, supporting medical necessity and accurate coding.

- **Pre-Authorization Processes:** Implement robust processes to verify insurance coverage and obtain necessary pre-authorizations prior to service delivery.

- **Timely Submission:** Develop internal controls to ensure claims are submitted within the payer's filing deadline, including checks for completeness and accuracy before submission.

Resolving Claim Denials

1. **Immediate Review and Response:** Promptly review and address denials, determining the root cause and necessary corrective action.

2. **Correct and Resubmit Claims:** Correct any errors identified in denied claims and resubmit them in accordance with payer guidelines.

3. **Appeal Incorrect Denials:** When appropriate, formally appeal denials by providing additional information or clarification to support the claim.

4. **Track and Monitor Appeals:** Maintain a system for tracking the status of appealed claims and document the outcomes for continuous learning and improvement.

Preventing Future Denials

- **Technology Solutions:** Utilize revenue cycle management software that includes claim scrubbing features to catch common errors before submission.

- **Collaboration with Clinical Staff:** Work closely with clinical staff to ensure that services are appropriately authorized, documented, and coded.

- **Payer Policy Updates:** Regularly review and stay informed about changes in payer policies and guidelines to adjust billing practices accordingly.

- **Continuous Improvement:** Use insights gained from denial analysis to implement process improvements, reducing the likelihood of future denials.

Conclusion

Effectively managing hospital claim denials is a multifaceted process that involves understanding the reasons behind denials, implementing strategies for resolution, and taking proactive steps to prevent future denials. By focusing on accurate documentation, coding, and adherence to payer policies, hospitals can improve their denial management processes, enhancing revenue integrity and financial stability. Continuous analysis, staff education, and leveraging technology are key components of a successful strategy to minimize claim denials and optimize hospital revenue cycle management.

16.4 Exercise: 10 MCQs with Answers at the End

Test your knowledge on hospital billing practices, focusing on inpatient vs. outpatient billing, understanding DRGs and inpatient coding, and managing hospital claim denials. This exercise is designed to reinforce key concepts and best practices in hospital billing.

Questions:

1. Inpatient billing is typically characterized by:

   A) DRG coding

   B) CPT/HCPCS coding

   C) Charging per service or procedure

   D) None of the above

2. Outpatient services are billed using:

   A) Global packages

   B) DRGs

   C) CPT/HCPCS codes

   D) Inpatient codes

3. One common reason for hospital claim denials is:

   A) Overpayment by insurance companies

   B) Lack of pre-authorization or referral

   C) Too few diagnosis codes

   D) Patient satisfaction

4. DRG stands for:

   A) Detailed Reimbursement Guide

   B) Diagnosis-Related Groups

   C) Direct Reimbursement Gains

   D) None of the above

5. Which of the following is true about managing hospital claim denials?

   A) It's best to ignore small denials as they cost more to appeal

   B) Denials should be analyzed to identify patterns

   C) Correcting and resubmitting claims is generally discouraged

   D) Appeals are rarely successful

6. The place of service (POS) code for telehealth services is:

   A) 11

   B) 02

   C) 22

D) 50

7. Observation services are billed as:

A) Inpatient services

B) Outpatient services

C) Neither, they are not billable

D) Both, depending on the duration of observation

8. A key strategy for preventing future claim denials is:

A) Reducing the amount of documentation

B) Utilizing revenue cycle management software

C) Ignoring payer policy updates

D) Increasing the number of services provided

9. The global surgical package includes all of the following EXCEPT:

A) Post-operative visits

B) Pre-operative visits within a certain timeframe

C) Procedures performed by another surgeon

D) The surgery itself

10. Accurate documentation in hospital billing is crucial for:

A) Speeding up the claim submission process only

B) Supporting medical necessity and accurate coding

C) Simplifying patient discharge instructions

D) Decreasing hospital readmission rates

Answers:

1. A) DRG coding

2. C) CPT/HCPCS codes

3. B) Lack of pre-authorization or referral

4. B) Diagnosis-Related Groups

5. B) Denials should be analyzed to identify patterns

6. B) 02

7. B) Outpatient services

8. B) Utilizing revenue cycle management software

9. C) Procedures performed by another surgeon

10. B) Supporting medical necessity and accurate coding

These questions and answers aim to deepen your understanding of hospital billing practices, highlighting the differences between inpatient and outpatient billing, the significance of DRGs in inpatient coding, and strategies for effectively managing hospital claim denials.

Chapter 17: Outsourcing Medical Billing

17.1 Pros and Cons of Outsourcing

Outsourcing medical billing involves hiring an external company to manage billing and coding processes, allowing healthcare providers to focus on patient care. While outsourcing can offer significant benefits, it's also important to consider potential drawbacks. Understanding the pros and cons of outsourcing medical billing can help healthcare practices make informed decisions that align with their operational goals and patient care standards.

Pros of Outsourcing Medical Billing

1. Increased Efficiency and Expertise:

   - Access to billing professionals with specialized knowledge and experience.

   - Reduced errors and improved compliance with coding regulations and payer policies.

2. Cost Savings:

- Potential reduction in overhead costs associated with staffing, training, and maintaining an in-house billing department.

- Variable costs instead of fixed, as many outsourcing companies charge a percentage of collections.

3. Focus on Patient Care:

- Allows healthcare providers to concentrate on clinical aspects and patient services by reducing administrative burdens.

- Can improve patient satisfaction by streamlining the billing process and reducing billing-related inquiries.

4. Scalability:

- Easier to scale operations with fluctuations in patient volume without the need to adjust staffing levels.

- Outsourced billing companies can handle increases in billing volume more readily.

5. Improved Cash Flow:

- Professional billing companies often ensure faster claim submission and follow-up, leading to improved collections and reduced days in accounts receivable (A/R).

Cons of Outsourcing Medical Billing

1. **Less Control:**

- Practices relinquish direct control over the billing process, relying on the outsourcing company to manage day-to-day operations.

- Potential challenges in maintaining the same level of oversight and immediacy in addressing billing issues.

2. **Concerns Over Patient Data Security:**

- Outsourcing involves sharing sensitive patient information with a third party, raising concerns about data privacy and security.

- Essential to ensure that the outsourcing company complies with HIPAA and other relevant regulations.

3. **Cost Considerations:**

- While outsourcing can be cost-effective, the fees charged by billing companies (usually a percentage of collections) may be higher than the cost of an efficient in-house team for some practices.

- Need to carefully evaluate the cost-benefit ratio and consider any additional fees for services like denial management or credentialing.

4. **Potential for Communication Issues:**

   - Risk of communication gaps between the healthcare provider and the billing company, which can affect billing accuracy and timeliness.

   - Important to establish clear communication channels and regular reporting practices.

5. **Dependency on Vendor:**

   - Developing a dependency on the outsourcing company, making it challenging to transition back to in-house billing if desired.

   - Risk of disruption in billing services during transitions between vendors.

Conclusion

Outsourcing medical billing can offer significant advantages, including cost savings, enhanced efficiency, and the ability to focus more on patient care. However, it's crucial to weigh these benefits against potential downsides like reduced control and concerns about data security. Each healthcare practice must consider its specific needs, volume, and resources when deciding whether to outsource medical billing or manage it in-house. Careful selection of a reputable and compliant billing company is essential to maximize the benefits of outsourcing while mitigating potential risks.

17.2 Selecting a Billing Service

Choosing the right medical billing service is a critical decision for healthcare providers aiming to outsource their billing operations. The effectiveness of the selected service can significantly impact a practice's financial health, compliance, and overall operational efficiency. Here are key considerations and steps to take when selecting a medical billing service.

Assess Your Practice's Needs

- **Volume and Specialty:** Consider the volume of billing and the specific needs of your medical specialty. Some billing services specialize in certain areas of healthcare and may be more adept at handling unique coding and billing challenges.

- **Service Scope:** Determine whether you need a comprehensive service that includes patient billing, insurance follow-up, and denial management, or if you're looking for assistance with specific aspects of the billing process.

Evaluate Potential Billing Services

1. **Experience and Reputation:**

   - Look for a billing service with a strong track record and experience in your healthcare sector. Check references and reviews from current and former clients to gauge satisfaction and performance.

2. Compliance and Security:

- Ensure the billing service is compliant with HIPAA and other relevant healthcare regulations. Inquire about their data security measures and procedures for protecting patient information.

3. Technology and Integration:

- Assess the billing service's technology platform. It should be capable of integrating with your existing electronic health record (EHR) system and practice management software to ensure seamless data exchange.

- Consider the ease of use and the reporting capabilities of their system.

4. Financial Terms and Transparency:

- Understand the billing service's fee structure. Most operate on a percentage basis, charging a portion of the collections. Compare rates and be wary of services with fees that are significantly lower or higher than average.

- Inquire about additional fees for services such as patient inquiries, postage, and setup costs.

5. Communication and Customer Service:

- Effective communication is crucial for a successful partnership. Evaluate the billing service's responsiveness and the availability of dedicated account managers.

- Assess their customer service approach, especially how they handle patient billing inquiries and disputes.

Request a Demonstration

- Before making a final decision, request a demonstration of the billing service's software and processes. This can provide insight into their efficiency, user-friendliness, and suitability for your practice.

Negotiate the Contract

- Once you've selected a billing service, carefully review the contract. Pay particular attention to terms regarding termination of the contract, service level agreements (SLAs), and confidentiality clauses.

- Consider involving a legal advisor to ensure that the contract meets your practice's needs and protects your interests.

Plan for Transition and Ongoing Evaluation

- Develop a plan for transitioning your billing operations to the service, including timelines, training, and data migration.

- Establish metrics for ongoing evaluation of the billing service's performance, including collection rates, denial rates, and turnaround times for claim processing.

Conclusion

Selecting the right medical billing service requires thorough research, careful consideration of your practice's needs, and clear communication about expectations. By choosing a partner that aligns with your operational goals and offers reliable, compliant, and efficient billing solutions, healthcare providers can enhance their revenue cycle management, allowing them to focus more on delivering quality patient care.

17.3 Managing the Transition

Transitioning to an outsourced medical billing service is a significant change for any healthcare practice. It involves shifting critical financial operations to an external partner, which can have far-reaching implications for your practice's workflow, financial health, and patient satisfaction. Effective management of this transition is crucial to minimize disruptions, maintain billing accuracy, and ensure a smooth handover. Here are key strategies to manage the transition effectively.

Prepare Thoroughly

- **Audit Current Billing Processes:** Conduct a comprehensive audit of your current billing processes to identify any issues or inefficiencies. This will help you understand what needs improvement and what expectations to set with the new billing service.

- **Communicate with Staff:** Inform your staff about the decision to outsource billing. Explain the reasons behind the move, how it will affect their daily tasks, and the benefits it will bring to the practice. Address any concerns and emphasize the positive impact on patient care and operational efficiency.

- **Select the Right Partner:** Ensure the billing service you choose is well-versed in your practice's specialty, compatible with your EHR and practice management systems, and has a solid track record of compliance and performance.

Establish Clear Communication Channels

- **Designate Points of Contact:** Assign specific individuals within your practice and at the billing service to serve as primary points of contact. This facilitates efficient communication and problem resolution.

- **Set Regular Meetings:** Schedule regular meetings with the billing service to discuss progress, review performance metrics, and address any issues. This keeps both parties aligned and fosters a collaborative relationship.

Ensure Data Compatibility and Integration

- **Data Migration:** Work closely with the billing service to ensure a smooth and accurate migration of patient data, billing records, and other essential information. Conduct thorough testing to verify data integrity.

- **System Integration:** Confirm that the billing service's software seamlessly integrates with your existing EHR and practice management systems. Integration is key to maintaining uninterrupted workflow and data exchange.

Train Your Team

- **Staff Training:** Provide training for your team on new procedures related to billing documentation, patient inquiries about billing, and how to interact with the billing service. Ensure everyone is comfortable with their role in the new workflow.

Monitor and Evaluate Performance

- **Define Key Performance Indicators (KPIs):** Establish clear metrics to evaluate the billing service's performance, including collection rates, denial rates, and turnaround times for claim processing.

- **Regular Reviews:** Conduct regular reviews of the billing service's performance against the agreed-upon KPIs. Use these reviews as opportunities to discuss improvements, adjustments, or any necessary corrective actions.

Maintain Oversight

- **Stay Engaged:** While outsourcing billing operations, it's crucial to maintain oversight. Ensure that billing practices align with your practice's standards and values, and remain involved in major billing decisions.

- **Patient Feedback:** Listen to patient feedback regarding billing and address any concerns promptly. Patient satisfaction with the billing process is a key indicator of the service's performance.

Conclusion

Managing the transition to an outsourced medical billing service requires careful planning, clear communication, and ongoing monitoring. By taking a proactive approach to each stage of the transition, healthcare practices can ensure a smooth shift that enhances billing efficiency, improves financial performance, and allows the practice to focus more on delivering quality patient care.

17.4 Exercise: 10 MCQs with Answers at the End

Test your understanding of outsourcing medical billing, including the pros and cons, selecting a billing service, and managing the transition to an outsourced provider. This exercise is designed to consolidate your knowledge and prepare you for implementing or improving outsourced billing processes in a healthcare setting.

Questions:

1. What is a primary advantage of outsourcing medical billing?

   A) Decreased control over billing processes

   B) Increased efficiency and expertise

   C) Higher costs due to outsourcing fees

   D) Less direct communication with patients

2. A key consideration when selecting a medical billing service is:

   A) The color scheme of their branding

   B) Their experience and reputation in the healthcare sector

   C) The number of employees they have

   D) Their office location

3. One potential drawback of outsourcing medical billing is:

A) Improved cash flow

B) Enhanced focus on patient care

C) Concerns over patient data security

D) Access to billing professionals

4. Effective communication during the transition to an outsourced billing service includes:

A) Ignoring staff concerns and questions

B) Designating points of contact and setting regular meetings

C) Limiting information to senior management only

D) Avoiding discussions about performance metrics

5. When managing the transition to outsourced billing, it's important to:

A) Disregard data migration accuracy

B) Reduce staff training to save costs

C) Ensure data compatibility and integration

D) Isolate the billing service from the rest of the practice

6. Regular reviews of the billing service's performance should focus on:

A) The color of their reports

B) Personal opinions rather than data

C) Key Performance Indicators (KPIs) agreed upon

D) The billing service's marketing efforts

7. A primary goal of staff training during a transition to an outsourced billing service is:

A) Decreasing staff morale

B) Increasing resistance to change

C) Ensuring comfort with new procedures

D) Ignoring the impact on daily tasks

8. System integration in outsourcing billing is crucial for:

A) Maintaining uninterrupted workflow and data exchange

B) Decreasing operational efficiency

C) Complicating the billing process

D) Limiting access to patient data

9. Monitoring and evaluating performance after outsourcing billing should:

   A) Be avoided to maintain a positive relationship with the billing service

   B) Occur once without any follow-up

   C) Include regular reviews and discussions on performance metrics

   D) Focus solely on financial aspects, ignoring patient satisfaction

10. Establishing clear communication channels with an outsourced billing service helps to:

   A) Increase misunderstandings and errors

   B) Facilitate efficient problem resolution

   C) Discourage staff from asking billing-related questions

   D) Limit the information flow to senior management

Answers:

1. B) Increased efficiency and expertise

2. B) Their experience and reputation in the healthcare sector

3. C) Concerns over patient data security

4. B) Designating points of contact and setting regular meetings

5. C) Ensure data compatibility and integration

6. C) Key Performance Indicators (KPIs) agreed upon

7. C) Ensuring comfort with new procedures

8. A) Maintaining uninterrupted workflow and data exchange

9. C) Include regular reviews and discussions on performance metrics

10. B) Facilitate efficient problem resolution

These questions and answers aim to enhance your understanding of the critical aspects of outsourcing medical billing, emphasizing the importance of selecting the right service, effectively managing the transition, and maintaining oversight to ensure the success of the outsourcing arrangement.

Chapter 18: Managing a Medical Billing Office

18.1 Office Setup and Staffing

Setting up and staffing a medical billing office requires careful planning and strategic decision-making to ensure efficient operations and optimal financial performance. A well-organized billing office is crucial for navigating the complexities of healthcare billing, maintaining compliance, and enhancing revenue cycle management. Here are key considerations for setting up and staffing your medical billing office.

Office Setup Considerations

1. **Infrastructure:** Ensure your office has the necessary infrastructure, including reliable internet, secure networking capabilities, and appropriate office equipment (computers, printers, scanners). Consider the layout to support efficient workflow and communication among staff.

2. **Software Systems:** Invest in robust medical billing and electronic health record (EHR) software that integrates seamlessly with payers and other healthcare systems. The software should support billing, coding, claim submission, follow-up, and reporting functionalities.

3. **Data Security and Compliance:** Implement strong data security measures to protect patient information and comply with HIPAA and other relevant regulations. This includes secure electronic transmission of data, encrypted storage solutions, and access controls.

4. **Disaster Recovery Plan:** Develop a comprehensive disaster recovery plan to protect data and ensure business continuity in case of emergencies, including data backup procedures and alternative work arrangements.

Staffing Considerations

1. **Roles and Responsibilities:** Define clear roles and responsibilities for your billing office staff. Common roles include billing specialists, coders, accounts receivable (A/R) specialists, and patient account representatives.

2. **Skills and Qualifications:** Look for candidates with specialized skills and qualifications in medical billing and coding, including familiarity with coding standards (ICD-10, CPT, HCPCS), payer policies, and billing software. Certifications from recognized organizations (e.g., AAPC, AHIMA) can be an indicator of proficiency.

3. **Training and Development:** Provide ongoing training and professional development opportunities for staff to stay

updated on the latest billing regulations, coding updates, and technology advancements.

4. **Team Structure:** Consider the size and volume of billing operations to determine the optimal team structure. A smaller practice may require a compact team that handles multiple aspects of billing, while larger operations might benefit from specialized roles focusing on specific areas (e.g., coding, denials management).

5. **Performance Monitoring:** Implement performance monitoring and evaluation systems to track productivity, accuracy, and efficiency. Use performance metrics to identify areas for improvement and recognize outstanding contributions.

Recruitment and Retention Strategies

1. **Competitive Compensation:** Offer competitive salaries and benefits to attract and retain skilled billing professionals. Consider performance-based incentives to motivate staff and improve performance.

2. **Positive Work Environment:** Foster a positive and supportive work environment that encourages teamwork, communication, and professional growth. Addressing staff feedback and concerns promptly can enhance job satisfaction and retention.

3. **Flexibility and Work-Life Balance:** Explore flexible working arrangements, such as telecommuting or flexible hours, to accommodate staff needs and promote work-life balance.

4. **Professional Development:** Support staff in obtaining further certifications and attending industry conferences or training sessions to advance their skills and knowledge.

Conclusion

Effectively setting up and staffing a medical billing office is foundational to successful revenue cycle management in healthcare. By focusing on the right infrastructure, technology, data security, and staff qualifications, practices can build a proficient billing team capable of managing billing processes efficiently, ensuring compliance, and maximizing revenue collection.

18.2 Effective Communication in the Office

Effective communication within a medical billing office is essential for maintaining a smooth workflow, ensuring accuracy in billing processes, and fostering a positive work environment. Given the complexity of medical billing and the need for collaboration across different roles, clear and open communication channels can significantly impact the office's overall efficiency and job satisfaction levels. Here are strategies to enhance communication in a medical billing office.

Establish Clear Communication Channels

- **Regular Meetings:** Schedule regular team meetings to discuss updates, share challenges, and brainstorm solutions. Include sessions for specific departments and whole-office meetings to ensure everyone is aligned with the office's goals and priorities.

- **Open-Door Policy:** Encourage an open-door policy where staff feel comfortable bringing their questions, concerns, and suggestions to management. This approach promotes transparency and trust.

- **Digital Communication Tools:** Utilize digital communication platforms (e.g., email, instant messaging apps, intranet systems) for daily updates and information sharing. Ensure these tools are used appropriately and maintain professionalism in digital communications.

Promote Team Collaboration

- **Cross-Functional Teams:** Create cross-functional teams for specific projects or problem-solving tasks. This encourages collaboration between different roles and departments, fostering a better understanding of each other's challenges and workflows.

- **Team Building Activities:** Organize team-building activities that are not directly related to work. These can help improve interpersonal relationships and communication among team members.

Implement Effective Training and Onboarding

- **Comprehensive Onboarding:** Develop a thorough onboarding program for new hires that includes an overview of communication protocols, key contacts, and how to access information. Pair new staff with experienced mentors for guidance.

- **Ongoing Training:** Offer regular training sessions on communication skills, conflict resolution, and teamwork. Encourage staff to attend external workshops or webinars that can enhance their communication abilities.

Encourage Feedback and Open Dialogue

- **Feedback Mechanisms:** Implement mechanisms for staff to provide feedback on processes, policies, and communication effectiveness. This could include suggestion boxes, anonymous surveys, or regular check-ins.

- **Address Conflicts Promptly:** Establish a clear process for addressing conflicts or misunderstandings in the workplace. Encourage open dialogue and seek to resolve issues constructively.

Recognize and Reward Effective Communication

- **Acknowledgment Programs:** Develop programs to acknowledge and reward staff members who demonstrate excellent communication skills or who contribute significantly to improving office communication.

- **Highlight Success Stories:** Share examples of effective communication leading to positive outcomes in staff meetings or newsletters. This can serve as motivation for others.

Ensure Consistency in Communication

- **Standard Operating Procedures (SOPs):** Create and maintain SOPs that include guidelines on communication practices within the office. Regularly review and update these procedures to reflect any changes or improvements.

- **Clear Role Definitions:** Ensure that everyone understands their role and responsibilities, including how they fit into the broader team and who they need to communicate with regularly.

Conclusion

Effective communication within a medical billing office not only enhances operational efficiency but also contributes to a more engaged and cohesive team. By establishing clear communication channels, promoting collaboration, encouraging open dialogue, and recognizing good communication practices, management can create a productive work environment conducive to achieving the office's billing and collection goals.

18.3 Workflow Management

Effective workflow management in a medical billing office is essential for optimizing operations, improving accuracy, and increasing the speed of revenue collection. By carefully designing and managing workflows, a billing office can minimize errors, reduce delays, and enhance overall productivity. Here are strategies to enhance workflow management in a medical billing office.

Assess and Map Current Workflows

- **Identify Key Processes:** Begin by identifying all critical billing processes, including patient registration, coding, claim submission, payment posting, and follow-up on denials and appeals.

- **Map Workflows:** Visually map out each process to understand the flow of tasks and identify any bottlenecks or redundancies that could be streamlined.

Implement Standard Operating Procedures (SOPs)

- **Develop SOPs:** Create detailed SOPs for each billing process based on best practices. SOPs should outline steps for completing tasks, roles and responsibilities, and compliance guidelines.

- **Regular Review and Updates:** Periodically review SOPs to incorporate changes in regulations, payer policies, and internal improvements. Ensure staff are trained on any updates.

Leverage Technology

- **Billing Software:** Utilize advanced medical billing software that supports automation of routine tasks, such as eligibility verification, claim scrubbing, and electronic claim submission.

- **Integration:** Ensure your billing software integrates seamlessly with EHR and practice management systems for efficient data exchange and reduced manual entry.

- **Analytics and Reporting:** Use software analytics to monitor workflow efficiency, identify trends in denials, and track key performance indicators (KPIs).

Optimize Task Allocation

- **Role Specialization:** Assign specific roles based on staff expertise and strengths. For example, have dedicated teams for coding, claim submission, and accounts receivable management.

- **Cross-Training:** Implement cross-training programs to create a flexible workforce capable of handling multiple aspects of the billing process, especially useful during peak periods or staff absences.

Continuous Improvement

- **Monitor Performance:** Regularly monitor the performance of billing processes through KPIs, such as claim denial rates, days in A/R, and collection ratios.

- **Feedback Loop:** Establish a feedback loop where staff can report issues, suggest improvements, and share best practices. Use this feedback to refine workflows continuously.

Focus on Communication and Collaboration

- **Internal Communication:** Foster open communication within the billing team and between the billing office and clinical staff to ensure clarity in billing requirements and quick resolution of coding or documentation questions.

- **Collaborative Problem-Solving:** Encourage a team approach to addressing workflow challenges, involving staff from various roles in brainstorming and implementing solutions.

Prioritize Training and Support

- **Ongoing Training:** Provide regular training for staff on billing regulations, coding updates, and new technologies to ensure they have the knowledge needed to manage their workflows effectively.

- **Supportive Environment:** Create a supportive work environment that recognizes the challenges of billing work and provides the necessary tools and resources to manage stress and prevent burnout.

Conclusion

Effective workflow management in a medical billing office is a dynamic process that requires ongoing assessment, the adoption of technology, strategic task allocation, and continuous improvement. By focusing on efficient processes, staff expertise, and open communication, billing offices can enhance productivity, improve accuracy, and accelerate revenue collection, ultimately contributing to the financial health of the healthcare practice.

18.4 Exercise: 10 MCQs with Answers at the End

Test your knowledge on managing a medical billing office, covering office setup and staffing, effective communication, and workflow management. This exercise aims to reinforce key principles for ensuring a productive and efficient billing office.

Questions:

1. What is the primary benefit of creating Standard Operating Procedures (SOPs) in a medical billing office?

   A) To reduce office space

   B) To ensure consistency and compliance in billing processes

   C) To increase the need for manual intervention

   D) To limit staff training opportunities

2. Effective use of medical billing software can:

   A) Increase manual data entry errors

   B) Reduce the efficiency of claim submissions

   C) Automate routine tasks and support analytics

   D) Decrease data security

3. Regular team meetings in a medical billing office are important for:

A) Discussing private patient information

B) Increasing bureaucracy and paperwork

C) Sharing updates and addressing challenges

D) Reducing team morale

4. Cross-training staff in a medical billing office helps to:

A) Create confusion among team members

B) Address staffing shortages and improve flexibility

C) Decrease staff competency in specific tasks

D) Isolate knowledge within individual roles

5. A primary goal of mapping out billing workflows is to:

A) Identify and eliminate efficient processes

B) Increase the complexity of billing operations

C) Identify bottlenecks and streamline operations

D) Discourage innovation and improvements

6. A key factor in selecting medical billing software is its ability to:

  A) Only handle small volumes of billing data

  B) Integrate with existing EHR and practice management systems

  C) Avoid generating reports and analytics

  D) Increase the time required for claim processing

7. Implementing an open-door policy in a billing office encourages:

  A) Staff to bypass formal communication channels

  B) Transparency and open communication

  C) Decreased trust among team members

  D) Limited feedback and suggestions

8. In managing a medical billing office, monitoring performance through KPIs helps to:

  A) Focus exclusively on financial metrics, ignoring operational efficiency

  B) Identify areas for improvement and track progress

  C) Discourage staff by focusing on negative outcomes

  D) Eliminate the need for staff training and development

9. The integration of billing software with EHR systems affects workflow management by:

A) Reducing the need for accurate documentation

B) Increasing manual data entry and the potential for errors

C) Enhancing data exchange and reducing duplicate entries

D) Isolating billing operations from clinical processes

10. The role specialization within a billing team is crucial for:

A) Decreasing the overall efficiency of the billing process

B) Ensuring tasks are assigned based on staff expertise and strengths

C) Encouraging staff to work in isolation

D) Limiting the scope of services the billing office can handle

Answers:

1. B) To ensure consistency and compliance in billing processes

2. C) Automate routine tasks and support analytics

3. C) Sharing updates and addressing challenges

4. B) Address staffing shortages and improve flexibility

5. C) Identify bottlenecks and streamline operations

6. B) Integrate with existing EHR and practice management systems

7. B) Transparency and open communication

8. B) Identify areas for improvement and track progress

9. C) Enhancing data exchange and reducing duplicate entries

10. B) Ensuring tasks are assigned based on staff expertise and strengths

These questions and answers aim to deepen your understanding of the strategic and operational considerations involved in managing a medical billing office, emphasizing the importance of SOPs, technology, communication, and team management in achieving efficiency and accuracy in billing processes.

Chapter 19: Professional Development in Medical Billing

19.1 Continuing Education and Certification

In the ever-evolving field of medical billing, continuing education and certification play crucial roles in professional development. Staying updated with the latest billing codes, regulations, and technologies is essential for maintaining accuracy in billing practices, ensuring compliance, and enhancing career prospects. This section explores the importance of continuing education and certification for professionals in medical billing.

Importance of Continuing Education

1. **Keeping Up with Changes:** The healthcare industry, including medical billing, is subject to frequent changes in regulations, payer policies, coding updates (ICD, CPT, HCPCS), and compliance requirements. Continuing education helps professionals stay informed about these changes, ensuring billing practices remain accurate and compliant.

2. **Enhancing Skills:** Ongoing education provides opportunities to deepen understanding of billing processes, improve problem-solving skills, and learn about new technologies and software in the field.

3. **Career Advancement:** Commitment to professional development can lead to career advancement opportunities, including higher-level positions, increased responsibilities, and salary growth.

Certification in Medical Billing

Certification demonstrates a professional's expertise and commitment to the field of medical billing. Several reputable organizations offer certifications for medical billing professionals, including:

- **AAPC (American Academy of Professional Coders):** Offers the Certified Professional Biller (CPB) certification, among others, focusing on the knowledge and skills needed for accurate medical billing.

- **AHIMA (American Health Information Management Association):** Offers credentials such as the Certified Coding Associate (CCA) and Certified Coding Specialist (CCS), relevant to professionals involved in medical billing and coding.

Benefits of Certification

- **Recognition of Expertise:** Certification acknowledges a professional's expertise and knowledge in medical billing, enhancing credibility with employers, colleagues, and clients.

- **Professional Growth:** Certified professionals often have access to a wider range of job opportunities, higher salaries, and greater career advancement potential.

- **Networking Opportunities:** Certification bodies often provide access to professional networks, forums, and resources, facilitating connections with peers and industry experts.

Pathways to Certification

1. **Education Requirements:** Most certification programs require candidates to have a certain level of education, such as a high school diploma or equivalent, and some may require completion of specific coursework related to medical billing and coding.

2. **Examination:** Certification typically involves passing a comprehensive examination that tests the candidate's knowledge of medical billing practices, coding, compliance, and insurance policies.

3. **Continuing Education:** To maintain certification, professionals are usually required to complete a certain number of continuing education units (CEUs) within a specified period, ensuring they stay current in the field.

Conclusion

Investing in continuing education and pursuing certification are pivotal steps for professionals in medical billing to enhance their knowledge, skills, and career prospects. These efforts not only benefit individual professionals but also contribute to the overall quality and efficiency of billing practices in healthcare, ultimately impacting patient satisfaction and financial stability.

19.2 Networking and Professional Associations

Networking and participation in professional associations are vital components of career development in medical billing. These activities provide opportunities for professionals to stay informed about industry trends, share best practices, and build relationships that can lead to career advancement and personal growth. Here's an overview of how networking and professional associations play a role in the field of medical billing.

Benefits of Networking

1. **Knowledge Sharing:** Networking allows medical billing professionals to exchange information on coding updates, regulatory changes, and innovative billing practices. This exchange can lead to improved accuracy and efficiency in billing processes.

2. **Career Opportunities:** Building a broad network can open doors to new job opportunities, collaborations, and partnerships. Networking events and professional association meetings are often where professionals learn about openings before they are widely advertised.

3. **Professional Support:** Networking provides a platform for professionals to seek advice, discuss challenges, and find solutions to common problems. This support can be invaluable in navigating the complexities of the medical billing field.

4. **Continuing Education:** Many networking groups and professional associations offer workshops, seminars, and conferences that count towards continuing education credits. These events keep professionals updated on industry standards and best practices.

Role of Professional Associations

Professional associations in medical billing serve as a hub for resources, education, and advocacy. They play a crucial role in advancing the profession and supporting the individual growth of their members.

Notable Associations in Medical Billing:

- **AAPC (American Academy of Professional Coders):** Offers certifications, continuing education, networking opportunities, and resources for coding and billing professionals.

- **AHIMA (American Health Information Management Association):** Focuses on health information management, including medical billing and coding, offering education, certification, and advocacy.

- **HBMA (Healthcare Business Management Association):** Dedicated to supporting the development of healthcare billing and management professionals through education, advocacy, and collaboration.

Getting Involved in Networking and Associations

1. **Membership:** Joining a professional association is a foundational step. Choose associations that align with your

career goals and offer valuable resources and networking opportunities.

2. **Conferences and Meetings:** Attend local, regional, and national conferences and meetings. These events are excellent opportunities to learn from industry leaders and connect with peers.

3. **Online Forums and Social Media:** Participate in online forums, LinkedIn groups, and other social media platforms related to medical billing. These digital platforms allow for networking and information sharing beyond geographical limitations.

4. **Volunteer and Leadership Roles:** Taking on volunteer or leadership roles within professional associations can significantly enhance your visibility in the field, develop your leadership skills, and expand your network.

Conclusion

Active networking and involvement in professional associations are crucial for career development in medical billing. These activities not only provide educational and career advancement opportunities but also foster a sense of community and support among professionals. By leveraging the resources and connections available through networking and associations, medical billing professionals can navigate their careers more effectively and contribute to the advancement of their field.

19.3 Career Advancement Strategies

Career advancement in medical billing requires a proactive approach, combining continuous learning, skill development, networking, and strategic career planning. By focusing on these areas, professionals can enhance their qualifications, increase their value to employers, and open up new career opportunities. Here are key strategies for advancing your career in medical billing.

Continuous Learning and Certification

- **Stay Updated:** Keep abreast of changes in healthcare regulations, coding updates, and billing practices. Subscribe to industry newsletters, attend webinars, and participate in relevant workshops and conferences.

- **Pursue Further Certifications:** Enhance your credentials by obtaining additional certifications from recognized organizations like AAPC (American Academy of Professional Coders) or AHIMA (American Health Information Management Association). Specialized certifications in areas like medical auditing, compliance, or practice management can broaden your skill set and make you more attractive to employers.

Networking and Professional Association Involvement

- **Build Professional Relationships:** Engage in networking by attending industry conferences, joining professional associations, and participating in online forums. Networking can lead to mentorship opportunities, collaborations, and job offers.

- **Contribute to the Field:** Share your knowledge and experiences by writing articles, speaking at events, or leading training sessions. This can raise your profile within the medical billing community and establish you as a thought leader.

Skill Enhancement

- **Develop Technical Skills:** Proficiency in medical billing software, EHR systems, and data analysis tools is crucial. Seek opportunities to learn new technologies and software that are emerging in the healthcare industry.

- **Enhance Soft Skills:** Communication, problem-solving, and customer service skills are vital in medical billing. Consider courses or training to develop these areas, as they can significantly impact your ability to advance into leadership roles.

Strategic Career Planning

- **Set Clear Career Goals:** Define your career objectives and create a roadmap to achieve them. Whether aiming for a management position, specializing in a certain area of billing, or transitioning into consulting, having clear goals can guide your professional development efforts.

- **Seek Out Mentorship:** Find a mentor who has achieved success in your desired career path. A mentor can provide guidance, advice, and support as you navigate your career advancement.

Performance Excellence

- **Demonstrate Value:** Excel in your current role by consistently delivering high-quality work, taking initiative to improve processes, and contributing positively to your team. Demonstrating your value can lead to recognition and advancement opportunities within your organization.

- **Document Achievements:** Keep a record of your achievements, including successful projects, process improvements, and positive feedback. This portfolio can be a powerful tool in performance reviews and job interviews.

Exploring New Opportunities

- **Consider Lateral Moves:** Sometimes, advancing your career may involve lateral moves to other departments or areas of specialization within medical billing. These moves can provide valuable experience and expose you to different aspects of the field.

- **Be Open to New Opportunities:** Whether it's a new project, a different role, or a job at another organization, be open to opportunities that align with your career goals and offer potential for growth.

Conclusion

Career advancement in medical billing is a multifaceted process that involves enhancing your skills, expanding your network, and strategically navigating your career path. By committing to continuous learning, seeking certifications, engaging in networking, and demonstrating excellence in your role, you can position yourself for success and achieve your professional aspirations in the dynamic field of medical billing.

19.4 Exercise: 10 MCQs with Answers at the End

Test your knowledge on professional development in medical billing, including continuing education, networking, and career advancement strategies. This exercise is designed to reinforce key concepts and strategies for advancing your career in the field of medical billing.

Questions:

1. Which organization offers the Certified Professional Biller (CPB) certification?

   A) AAPC

   B) AHIMA

C) HBMA

D) AMA

2. Continuous learning in medical billing is important for:

A) Keeping up with changes in healthcare regulations and coding updates

B) Reducing the need for networking

C) Limiting career advancement opportunities

D) Decreasing operational efficiency

3. Effective networking can lead to:

A) Decreased knowledge sharing

B) Fewer career opportunities

C) Professional support and mentorship

D) Increased data security risks

4. Enhancing soft skills in medical billing is beneficial for:

A) Only entry-level positions

B) Advancing into leadership roles

C) Reducing work efficiency

D) Limiting job responsibilities

5. Setting clear career goals in medical billing can:

   A) Discourage professional growth

   B) Guide your professional development efforts

   C) Increase job dissatisfaction

   D) Decrease work-life balance

6. Participating in professional associations can provide:

   A) Limited networking opportunities

   B) Access to continuing education and resources

   C) Decreased industry knowledge

   D) Fewer job prospects

7. Developing technical skills in medical billing is crucial for:

   A) Only working with paper records

   B) Proficiency in billing software and EHR systems

   C) Avoiding career advancement

   D) Decreasing accuracy in billing processes

8. Mentorship in medical billing can offer:

   A) Guidance and support in navigating your career

   B) Decreased professional network size

   C) Limited access to industry insights

D) Reduced professional confidence

9. Demonstrating value in your current role can lead to:

A) Recognition and advancement opportunities

B) Increased job insecurity

C) Ignored achievements

D) A static career path

10. Strategic career planning involves:

A) Avoiding setting specific career objectives

B) Ignoring changes in the healthcare industry

C) Defining your career objectives and creating a roadmap to achieve them

D) Limiting professional development to in-house training only

Answers:

1. A) AAPC

2. A) Keeping up with changes in healthcare regulations and coding updates

3. C) Professional support and mentorship

4. B) Advancing into leadership roles

5. B) Guide your professional development efforts

6. B) Access to continuing education and resources

7. B) Proficiency in billing software and EHR systems

8. A) Guidance and support in navigating your career

9. A) Recognition and advancement opportunities

10. C) Defining your career objectives and creating a roadmap to achieve them

These questions and answers aim to highlight the importance of ongoing education, networking, and strategic planning in advancing a career in medical billing. By engaging in these activities, professionals can enhance their skills, expand their professional network, and navigate their career path more effectively.

Chapter 20: Technological Advances in Medical Billing

20.1 Emerging Technologies in Healthcare

The landscape of healthcare, particularly in medical billing and revenue cycle management, is rapidly evolving with the advent of new technologies. These advancements aim to increase efficiency, reduce errors, and enhance the overall patient experience. Understanding these technologies and their potential impact is crucial for professionals in the field. Here's an overview of some key emerging technologies reshaping healthcare.

Artificial Intelligence (AI) and Machine Learning (ML)

- **Automated Coding and Billing:** AI algorithms can assist in automating the coding process, reducing manual entry errors, and ensuring more accurate billing.

- **Predictive Analytics:** ML models can analyze historical data to predict trends such as potential claim denials, helping practices proactively address issues before they impact revenue.

- **Chatbots for Patient Interaction:** AI-powered chatbots can handle patient inquiries about billing and insurance coverage, improving communication and patient satisfaction.

Blockchain Technology

- **Secure Data Exchange:** Blockchain can facilitate secure, tamper-proof data exchange between healthcare providers, payers, and patients, enhancing privacy and trust in the billing process.

- **Smart Contracts:** These can automate and streamline contract management and compliance with payer agreements, reducing administrative overhead and disputes.

Electronic Health Records (EHR) Integration

- **Enhanced Data Accuracy:** Seamless integration between EHR systems and billing software ensures that patient data and treatment details are accurately reflected in billing documents, minimizing discrepancies and denials.

- **Real-time Eligibility Checks:** EHR integration allows for real-time insurance eligibility verification, reducing the likelihood of billing errors due to coverage issues.

Telehealth and Remote Patient Monitoring

- **Expansion of Billing Opportunities:** As telehealth services become more prevalent, billing systems are adapting to include telehealth-specific coding and reimbursement strategies.

- **Remote Patient Monitoring (RPM) Billing:** RPM services offer new billing opportunities and require an understanding of emerging codes and reimbursement policies.

Interoperability Standards

- **Streamlined Data Sharing:** Adoption of interoperability standards facilitates smoother data exchange across different healthcare systems, improving the efficiency of billing processes and reducing delays.

Cloud-based Billing Solutions

- **Accessibility and Scalability:** Cloud-based medical billing software offers greater accessibility, allowing billing staff to work remotely while ensuring data security. It also scales easily to accommodate growing practices.

Mobile Payments and Online Billing Portals

- **Patient Convenience:** Offering mobile payment options and online billing portals aligns with consumer preferences for digital interactions, potentially speeding up collections and improving patient satisfaction.

Impact of Technological Advances

- **Operational Efficiency:** Emerging technologies can automate routine tasks, allowing billing staff to focus on more complex issues and strategic initiatives.

- **Compliance and Accuracy:** Technology aids in maintaining compliance with ever-changing regulations and ensures higher accuracy in billing and coding.

- **Patient Engagement:** Enhanced communication tools and digital payment options improve the patient experience and engagement with the billing process.

Conclusion

The integration of emerging technologies into medical billing processes represents a significant shift towards more efficient, accurate, and patient-centered healthcare. By staying informed about these advancements and embracing relevant technologies, billing professionals can ensure their practices remain competitive, compliant, and financially healthy in the evolving healthcare landscape.

20.2 Integrating New Technology into Billing

Integrating new technology into medical billing processes is essential for practices looking to improve efficiency, accuracy, and patient satisfaction. However, successful integration requires careful planning, training, and adjustment to workflows. Here are steps and considerations for effectively integrating new technology into your medical billing operations.

Assessment and Planning

1. **Identify Needs:** Begin by assessing your current billing processes to identify areas that could benefit from new technology, such as automation of routine tasks, enhanced data analytics, or improved patient communication.

2. **Research Solutions:** Explore technology solutions that address your identified needs. Consider options like AI-enhanced billing software, blockchain for secure data exchange, or integrated EHR systems.

3. **Evaluate Vendors:** Assess potential technology vendors based on their reputation, support services, compliance with healthcare regulations, and the ability to integrate with your existing systems.

4. **Cost-Benefit Analysis:** Conduct a cost-benefit analysis to determine the potential return on investment (ROI) of integrating new technology. Consider both direct costs and indirect benefits, such as time savings and improved claim acceptance rates.

Implementation

1. **Develop an Implementation Plan:** Create a detailed plan outlining the timeline, key milestones, and responsibilities for integrating the new technology. Ensure the plan includes data migration strategies, testing phases, and contingency plans.

2. **Engage Stakeholders:** Involve key stakeholders, including billing staff, IT personnel, and management, in the planning and implementation process. Their input can provide valuable insights and help ensure buy-in.

3. **Training and Support:** Provide comprehensive training for all users on the new technology, focusing on how it changes existing workflows and improves billing processes. Ensure ongoing support is available to address any questions or issues.

Testing and Evaluation

1. **Pilot Testing:** Initially, conduct pilot testing with a small group of users or for a subset of billing processes. This allows you to identify and resolve any issues before full-scale implementation.

2. **Monitor Performance:** After implementation, closely monitor the technology's performance against predefined metrics, such as error rates, billing cycle times, and patient satisfaction. Use this data to make adjustments as needed.

3. **Gather Feedback:** Collect feedback from users to understand their experiences with the new technology. This feedback can inform future training, support, and possibly further technological enhancements.

Ongoing Optimization

1. **Continuous Improvement:** View the integration of new technology as an ongoing process. Regularly review and update your technology solutions to adapt to changing healthcare regulations, billing practices, and advancements in technology.

2. **Stay Informed:** Keep abreast of emerging technologies and industry trends that could further enhance your billing processes. Engage with professional networks, attend industry conferences, and participate in relevant training sessions.

3. **Evaluate Impact:** Periodically assess the impact of the integrated technology on your billing operations and overall practice performance. This evaluation should consider financial metrics, operational efficiency, staff satisfaction, and patient engagement.

Conclusion

Integrating new technology into medical billing processes can significantly enhance operational efficiency, accuracy, and patient experience. Successful integration requires careful planning, stakeholder engagement, comprehensive training, and ongoing evaluation. By adopting a strategic approach to technology integration, medical billing offices can ensure they remain competitive and responsive to the evolving healthcare landscape.

20.3 The Future of Medical Billing

The future of medical billing is poised for transformative changes driven by technological advancements, regulatory shifts, and evolving healthcare delivery models. These changes aim to streamline billing processes, improve accuracy, enhance patient engagement, and ultimately lead to more efficient and patient-centric healthcare systems. Here's a glimpse into the future trends and developments in medical billing.

Increased Automation and AI Integration

- **Smart Automation:** The use of AI and machine learning will become more prevalent in automating routine tasks such as data entry, claim submission, and follow-up on unpaid claims. This will reduce manual errors and free up staff to focus on more complex billing issues.

- **Predictive Analytics:** AI-driven predictive analytics will play a significant role in identifying potential claim denials before submission, enabling preemptive corrections and improving the claims acceptance rate.

Blockchain for Secure Data Management

- **Enhanced Security and Transparency:** Blockchain technology will increasingly be used for secure and transparent data management, facilitating trust and efficiency in the exchange of medical records, billing information, and payment transactions between healthcare providers, payers, and patients.

Interoperability and Seamless Data Exchange

- **Unified Health Records:** The push for interoperability among EHR systems will intensify, leading to seamless data exchange across different healthcare providers and billing systems. This will simplify the billing process for services delivered by multiple providers and ensure more accurate billing based on comprehensive patient records.

Telehealth and Remote Services Billing

- **Standardized Telehealth Billing:** As telehealth continues to grow, standardized coding and billing guidelines for remote and virtual health services will become established. This will include clear reimbursement policies for telehealth across all payers, ensuring consistent revenue streams for providers offering remote care.

Patient-Centric Billing Experiences

- **Transparent Pricing and Payment Options:** There will be a shift towards more transparent pricing and flexible payment options, driven by consumer demand and regulatory requirements. Patients will have access to clear cost estimates before services are rendered and user-friendly payment portals to manage their healthcare expenses.

- **Personalized Communication:** Advanced CRM (Customer Relationship Management) systems will enable personalized communication with patients regarding their billing and insurance queries, enhancing patient satisfaction and engagement.

Regulatory and Compliance Evolution

- **Adaptation to New Regulations:** Ongoing changes in healthcare regulations will require billing processes to be highly adaptable. Billing offices will need to stay informed and quickly adjust to new compliance requirements, reimbursement models, and reporting standards.

- **Value-Based Care and Billing:** As the healthcare industry continues to move towards value-based care, billing processes will evolve to accommodate new reimbursement models based on patient outcomes, quality of care, and cost efficiency.

Enhanced Professional Development Opportunities

- **Skill Development:** The increasing complexity and technological orientation of medical billing will create demand for professionals with advanced skills in data analytics, IT, and customer service, alongside traditional billing expertise.

- **Continuing Education:** There will be a greater emphasis on continuing education and professional certification to keep billing staff updated on the latest trends, technologies, and regulatory changes.

Conclusion

The future of medical billing is characterized by technological innovation, regulatory adaptation, and a shift towards more patient-centered approaches. By embracing these changes, medical billing professionals can look forward to a future where billing processes are more streamlined, accurate, and integrated with the overall goal of improving healthcare delivery and patient outcomes.

20.4 Exercise: 10 MCQs with Answers at the End

Test your understanding of the technological advances in medical billing, including emerging technologies, integration strategies, and future trends. This exercise is designed to reinforce your knowledge of how technology is shaping the future of medical billing.

Questions:

1. Which technology is predicted to automate routine tasks in medical billing?

   A) Blockchain

   B) Artificial Intelligence (AI)

   C) Fax machines

   D) Manual ledgers

2. Blockchain technology in medical billing enhances:

   A) Error rates in coding

   B) Transparency and data security

   C) Paper-based recordkeeping

   D) Complexity in claim submission

3. Interoperability in healthcare systems aims to:

   A) Reduce data sharing between systems

   B) Increase manual data entry requirements

   C) Facilitate seamless data exchange

   D) Isolate patient records within single providers

4. Predictive analytics can help medical billing by:

A) Decreasing the accuracy of billing

B) Identifying potential claim denials before submission

C) Ignoring historical data trends

D) Increasing the volume of denied claims

5. Telehealth billing in the future will likely:

A) Remain an undefined area without clear guidelines

B) See standardized coding and reimbursement policies

C) Exclude remote patient monitoring

D) Reduce in prevalence and importance

6. Patient-centric billing experiences emphasize:

A) Increased opacity in pricing

B) Limited payment options

C) Transparent pricing and flexible payment options

D) Automated responses without personalization

7. The move towards value-based care will require billing processes to adapt to:

A) Fixed reimbursement models regardless of care quality

B) Reimbursement models based on patient outcomes and cost efficiency

C) Solely the volume of patients treated

D) Traditional fee-for-service models without innovation

8. AI-driven predictive analytics in medical billing primarily aim to:

A) Simplify patient care procedures

B) Predict and improve weather forecasting

C) Enhance the speed of manual coding

D) Improve claims acceptance rates by preemptive corrections

9. The integration of new technology into medical billing processes requires:

A) Ignoring staff training and support

B) Comprehensive planning, including data migration and user training

C) Sole reliance on outdated software systems

D) Decreased focus on data security and compliance

10. Future professional development in medical billing will likely focus on skills in:

   A) Typewriter maintenance

   B) Data analytics, IT, and customer service

   C) Morse code proficiency

   D) 20th-century filing techniques

Answers:

1. B) Artificial Intelligence (AI)

2. B) Transparency and data security

3. C) Facilitate seamless data exchange

4. B) Identifying potential claim denials before submission

5. B) See standardized coding and reimbursement policies

6. C) Transparent pricing and flexible payment options

7. B) Reimbursement models based on patient outcomes and cost efficiency

8. D) Improve claims acceptance rates by preemptive corrections

9. B) Comprehensive planning, including data migration and user training

10. B) Data analytics, IT, and customer service

These questions highlight the significant impact of emerging technologies on the future of medical billing, emphasizing the importance of staying informed and adapting to technological advancements to enhance billing processes, improve efficiency, and meet the evolving needs of the healthcare industry.

Chapter 21: Customer Service in Medical Billing

21.1 Principles of Excellent Customer Service

In the context of medical billing, customer service plays a pivotal role in patient satisfaction and retention. Excellent customer service in this field goes beyond mere transactional interactions; it involves providing clear, compassionate, and timely communication about billing processes and charges. Here are the core principles of delivering excellent customer service in medical billing.

Clear Communication

- **Transparency:** Provide clear and straightforward explanations of billing processes, charges, and payment options. Transparency helps in building trust and reducing confusion.

- **Proactive Information:** Inform patients about potential costs upfront, including estimates for services and procedures, to avoid surprise billing issues.

Empathy and Understanding

- **Compassionate Interactions:** Approach each patient interaction with empathy, recognizing that discussions about billing can be stressful. Show understanding and willingness to find solutions that meet patients' needs.

- **Personalized Service:** Tailor communication and payment options to individual patient situations, acknowledging that each patient's financial situation and concerns are unique.

Responsiveness

- **Prompt Responses:** Ensure inquiries and concerns are addressed promptly. A quick response time can significantly impact patient satisfaction and reduce frustration.

- **Follow-up:** Implement follow-up procedures to ensure that patient questions have been fully resolved and that they understand their billing statements and payment responsibilities.

Accuracy

- **Billing Accuracy:** Strive for precision in all billing statements to prevent errors that can lead to disputes and dissatisfaction. Regular audits and checks can help maintain accuracy.

- **Correction of Errors:** When errors occur, correct them swiftly and inform the patient of any changes to their billing statement or account.

Patient Education

- **Understanding of Insurance Benefits:** Educate patients on how to understand their insurance benefits, coverage, and potential out-of-pocket costs. This can empower patients and reduce billing-related inquiries.

- **Billing Policies and Procedures:** Clearly explain your practice's billing policies, including payment options, timelines, and procedures for disputing charges or requesting financial assistance.

Flexibility

- **Payment Options:** Offer flexible payment plans and options to accommodate patients' financial situations, reducing the financial burden and fostering goodwill.

- **Dispute Resolution:** Have clear, fair processes in place for resolving billing disputes. Being open to negotiation and compromise can help maintain positive patient relationships.

Feedback Mechanism

- **Soliciting Feedback:** Actively seek feedback from patients regarding their billing experience. This can provide valuable insights into areas for improvement.

- **Continuous Improvement:** Use patient feedback to continually refine and improve billing processes and customer service practices.

Training and Empowerment

- **Staff Training:** Regularly train billing staff on customer service best practices, including communication skills, empathy, and handling difficult conversations.

- **Empowerment:** Empower staff to make decisions and take actions that improve patient satisfaction, within established guidelines.

Conclusion

Excellent customer service in medical billing is about more than just collecting payments; it's about fostering trust, understanding, and satisfaction among patients. By adhering to these principles, medical billing professionals can enhance the patient experience, reduce complaints, and build a positive reputation for their practice or healthcare organization.

21.2 Handling Difficult Situations

In medical billing, encountering difficult situations and conversations with patients regarding billing issues is inevitable. Handling these situations with professionalism, empathy, and effective communication can turn potentially negative experiences into positive outcomes. Here are strategies for managing challenging scenarios in medical billing.

Listen Actively

- **Understand the Concern:** Give patients the opportunity to express their concerns without interruption. Active listening helps in understanding the root cause of the issue.

- **Acknowledge Feelings:** Recognize and validate the patient's feelings. A simple acknowledgment can diffuse tension and show that you are taking their concerns seriously.

Maintain Professionalism

- **Stay Calm:** Keep a calm and professional demeanor, even if the patient becomes upset or angry. Your tone and attitude can significantly influence the direction of the conversation.

- **Use Clear, Respectful Language:** Avoid using jargon that might confuse patients. Be respectful and clear in your communication, aiming to explain billing issues in terms that are easy to understand.

Provide Clear Explanations

- **Explain Billing Processes:** Often, frustration arises from a lack of understanding. Clearly explain the billing process, including how charges are determined, how insurance coverage is applied, and why the patient may owe a balance.

- **Discuss Specific Issues:** Address the patient's specific concerns directly, providing detailed explanations and pointing out any misunderstandings or errors.

Offer Solutions

- **Flexible Payment Options:** If the dispute involves an inability to pay, discuss available payment plans or financial assistance programs that may alleviate the patient's burden.

- **Correct Mistakes Promptly:** If an error on the billing statement is identified, correct it immediately and inform the patient of the correction and any resulting changes to their balance.

Seek Resolution

- **Work Towards a Solution:** Aim to find a solution that addresses the patient's concerns while staying within the policies of your billing office or healthcare organization.

- **Agree on Next Steps:** Once a resolution is reached, clearly outline the next steps, whether it's a revised billing statement, setting up a payment plan, or submitting additional information to insurance.

Follow Up

- **Confirm Resolution:** After the initial conversation, follow up with the patient to ensure that the agreed-upon actions have been completed and that they are satisfied with the resolution.

- **Document the Interaction:** Keep detailed records of the conversation, the patient's concerns, the solutions offered, and the outcome. This documentation can be valuable for future reference and for improving billing practices.

Use Difficult Situations as Learning Opportunities

- **Identify Trends:** Analyze difficult situations to identify common issues or trends that may indicate a need for changes in billing practices or patient communication strategies.

- **Continuous Improvement:** Use insights gained from handling difficult situations to improve billing processes, enhance customer service training, and prevent similar issues in the future.

Conclusion

Handling difficult situations in medical billing requires a combination of empathy, clear communication, problem-solving, and a commitment to fairness and professionalism. By adopting these strategies, billing professionals can navigate challenging conversations effectively, maintain positive patient relationships, and contribute to the overall reputation and success of their healthcare organization.

21.3 Improving Patient Satisfaction

Improving patient satisfaction within the context of medical billing is crucial for healthcare organizations. Positive billing experiences can significantly impact overall patient satisfaction, loyalty, and the likelihood of patients recommending the healthcare provider to others. Here are key strategies to enhance patient satisfaction in medical billing.

Transparent and Proactive Communication

- **Upfront Cost Estimates:** Provide patients with clear estimates of their expected charges before services are rendered, helping to manage expectations and reduce billing surprises.

- **Insurance Benefits and Coverage Explanation:** Assist patients in understanding their insurance coverage, including what is covered, their deductibles, copayments, and any out-of-pocket costs they may incur.

- **Billing Statements Clarity:** Ensure billing statements are straightforward and easy to understand. Include detailed explanations of charges and a glossary of billing terms if necessary.

Personalized Billing Support

- **Dedicated Support Staff:** Offer access to dedicated billing support staff who can answer questions, resolve issues, and guide patients through the billing process.

- **Patient Portals:** Utilize patient portals that allow patients to view their billing statements, make payments, set up payment plans, and communicate with billing support online.

Flexible Payment Options

- **Payment Plans:** Provide flexible payment plans for patients who cannot pay their bills in full. Clearly communicate the terms and conditions of these plans.

- **Multiple Payment Methods:** Accept various payment methods, including online payments, credit cards, checks, and mobile payment platforms, to make it convenient for patients to settle their bills.

Timely and Responsive Service

- **Prompt Billing:** Issue billing statements promptly after services are rendered to keep charges fresh in patients' minds and reduce confusion.

- **Efficient Issue Resolution:** Ensure billing inquiries and disputes are addressed and resolved quickly. A responsive billing service can significantly enhance patient satisfaction.

Patient Education

- **Billing Processes:** Educate patients about the billing process, including how claims are processed, how payments are applied, and how to read their billing statements.

- **Financial Responsibility:** Clearly communicate patients' financial responsibilities, including copays and deductibles, and educate them on how to avoid common billing issues.

Feedback Mechanism

- **Solicit Feedback:** Actively seek feedback from patients regarding their billing experience. This can be done through surveys, suggestion boxes, or during follow-up calls.

- **Continuous Improvement:** Use patient feedback to identify areas of improvement and implement changes to billing practices, policies, and patient communication strategies.

Invest in Staff Training

- **Customer Service Training:** Provide regular customer service training for billing staff, focusing on empathy, communication skills, and effective problem-solving techniques.

- **Billing Accuracy Training:** Emphasize the importance of billing accuracy and compliance in training programs to reduce billing errors and disputes.

Conclusion

Improving patient satisfaction in medical billing requires a multifaceted approach that emphasizes transparency, personalized support, flexibility, and responsiveness. By implementing these strategies, healthcare organizations can create positive billing experiences that contribute to overall patient satisfaction and loyalty, thereby enhancing the reputation and success of the healthcare provider.

21.4 Exercise: 10 MCQs with Answers at the End

Test your knowledge on customer service in medical billing, covering principles of excellent customer service, handling difficult situations, and strategies for improving patient satisfaction. This exercise is designed to reinforce important concepts and practices for enhancing the patient experience in medical billing.

Questions:

1. What is essential for providing clear communication in medical billing?

   A) Using complex medical jargon

   B) Transparency and straightforward explanations

C) Providing minimal information to avoid questions

D) Delaying the delivery of billing statements

2. Empathy in medical billing customer service is important for:

   A) Only patients who are upset

   B) Building trust and understanding with all patients

   C) Decreasing the efficiency of the billing process

   D) Making billing processes more complex

3. When handling difficult billing situations, it's crucial to:

   A) Escalate the situation immediately

   B) Listen actively and acknowledge the patient's feelings

   C) Ignore patient feedback

   D) Focus solely on policy enforcement without flexibility

4. Offering flexible payment options is a strategy to:

   A) Increase patient confusion

   B) Improve patient satisfaction by accommodating financial situations

   C) Discourage timely payments

   D) Simplify billing processes for the billing office

5. Proactive communication about potential costs and insurance coverage helps to:

A) Reduce transparency in billing

B) Manage patient expectations and reduce surprises

C) Increase the number of billing disputes

D) Complicate the patient's understanding of their charges

6. Dedicated billing support staff contribute to patient satisfaction by:

A) Limiting access to billing information

B) Providing personalized assistance and resolving issues

C) Increasing response times to inquiries

D) Focusing on the needs of the billing office over patients

7. The use of patient portals in medical billing enhances patient satisfaction by offering:

A) Less control over their billing and payment options

B) Online access to billing statements and payment features

C) Reduced communication channels with billing staff

D) Increased complexity in managing their healthcare expenses

8. Timely and responsive service in medical billing involves:

A) Delaying the issuance of billing statements

B) Slow responses to billing inquiries and disputes

C) Prompt billing and efficient issue resolution

D) Avoiding follow-up on unresolved billing issues

9. Patient education on billing processes and financial responsibility can:

A) Decrease patient satisfaction

B) Empower patients and reduce billing-related inquiries

C) Lead to more billing errors and disputes

D) Make the billing process less transparent

10. Continuous improvement in medical billing customer service is achieved through:

A) Ignoring patient feedback

B) Regularly seeking and acting on patient feedback

C) Maintaining the status quo in billing practices

D) Decreasing the flexibility of payment options

Answers:

1. B) Transparency and straightforward explanations

2. B) Building trust and understanding with all patients

3. B) Listen actively and acknowledge the patient's feelings

4. B) Improve patient satisfaction by accommodating financial situations

5. B) Manage patient expectations and reduce surprises

6. B) Providing personalized assistance and resolving issues

7. B) Online access to billing statements and payment features

8. C) Prompt billing and efficient issue resolution

9. B) Empower patients and reduce billing-related inquiries

10. B) Regularly seeking and acting on patient feedback

These questions and answers aim to highlight the importance of clear communication, empathy, flexibility, and responsiveness in delivering excellent customer service in medical billing. By adopting these practices, billing professionals can significantly enhance patient satisfaction and contribute positively to the overall patient experience.

Chapter 22: Financial Policy and Management

22.1 Developing a Financial Policy

A well-defined financial policy is crucial for any healthcare organization or medical practice. It sets clear expectations for patients regarding payments and billing, and it establishes guidelines for the practice's staff on managing financial transactions. A comprehensive financial policy can reduce billing errors, improve cash flow, and enhance patient satisfaction by providing transparency. Here are steps and considerations for developing an effective financial policy.

Understand Legal and Ethical Requirements

- **Compliance:** Ensure your financial policy complies with all applicable laws and regulations, including those related to billing, debt collection, and patient privacy.

- **Ethics:** The policy should also reflect ethical considerations, treating patients fairly and with respect, especially in cases of financial hardship.

Define Payment Expectations

- **Payment Timing:** Clearly state when payments are expected, such as at the time of service for copays or within a certain number of days post-billing for balances.

- **Accepted Payment Methods:** Specify which forms of payment your practice accepts (e.g., cash, checks, credit cards, online payments).

Outline Insurance Billing Practices

- **Insurance Verification:** Describe the process for verifying patient insurance coverage and the patient's responsibility for ensuring their insurance information is up to date.

- **Claims Submission:** Explain how insurance claims are submitted, including timelines and the process for handling denied claims or appeals.

Detail Patient Responsibilities

- **Understanding Benefits:** Encourage patients to understand their insurance benefits and inform them of their responsibility for charges not covered by insurance.

- **Providing Accurate Information:** Emphasize the importance of patients providing accurate personal and insurance information.

Address Financial Assistance and Payment Plans

- **Assistance Programs:** If your practice offers financial assistance or sliding scale fees for qualifying patients, include details about eligibility and how to apply.

- **Payment Plans:** Outline the availability of payment plans, including how patients can set them up, terms, and conditions.

Explain the Collections Process

- **Delinquent Accounts:** Clearly describe the steps the practice takes when an account becomes delinquent, including any fees, interest, or third-party collection involvement.

- **Dispute Resolution:** Provide a process for patients to dispute charges they believe are incorrect, including contact information and expected resolution timelines.

Communicate the Policy to Patients

- **Policy Distribution:** Distribute the financial policy to new patients and make it available on your website. Consider requiring patients to sign an acknowledgment form indicating they have read and understand the policy.

- **Staff Training:** Train your staff on the details of the financial policy so they can answer patient questions accurately and consistently.

Review and Update Regularly

- **Ongoing Evaluation:** Regularly review and update the financial policy to reflect changes in healthcare regulations, insurance practices, and your own operational procedures.

- **Feedback Incorporation:** Use feedback from patients and staff to identify areas of the policy that may need clarification or adjustment.

Conclusion

Developing a comprehensive financial policy is a critical step for healthcare providers in managing their financial interactions with patients. By clearly outlining payment responsibilities, insurance practices, and available financial assistance, practices can foster a transparent and fair environment. This not only helps in minimizing billing disputes and enhancing cash flow but also contributes to building trust and satisfaction among patients.

22.2 Managing Accounts Receivable

Managing accounts receivable (A/R) effectively is crucial for maintaining the financial health of any healthcare practice. Accounts receivable represent the money owed to the practice for services provided but not yet paid. Efficient A/R management ensures timely collection of payments, improves cash flow, and reduces the risk of bad debt. Here are strategies to manage accounts receivable effectively.

1. Accurate Billing and Coding

- **Ensure Accuracy:** Minimize errors in billing and coding to reduce claim denials and delays in payments. Use automated billing software with claim scrubbing features to catch common errors before submission.

- **Stay Updated:** Keep up with changes in coding standards and payer policies to ensure claims are compliant and accurately reflect the services provided.

2. Efficient Claim Submission

- **Timely Submission:** Submit claims to insurance companies as soon as possible after services are rendered to expedite payment.

- **Follow Up:** Regularly follow up on outstanding claims to check their status and resolve any issues that may be delaying payment.

3. Proactive Patient Communication

- **Clear Financial Policies:** Communicate your financial policies to patients upfront, including payment expectations and procedures for handling unpaid balances.

- **Patient Statements:** Send clear and understandable patient statements promptly. Include itemized charges, payments received, and the balance due.

4. Monitoring and Reporting

- **A/R Aging Reports:** Regularly review accounts receivable aging reports to identify and prioritize overdue accounts. Take action on accounts that are past due based on the age of the receivable.

- **Key Performance Indicators (KPIs):** Monitor KPIs such as Days in A/R, Collection Rate, and Denial Rate to assess the effectiveness of your A/R management practices.

5. Payment Plans and Financial Assistance

- **Offer Payment Plans:** For patients who cannot pay their balances in full, offer reasonable payment plans that allow them to pay over time while securing revenue for the practice.

- **Financial Assistance:** Clearly communicate any financial assistance programs available to help patients with financial hardships.

6. Effective Follow-Up on Delinquent Accounts

- **Structured Follow-Up Process:** Implement a structured process for following up on delinquent accounts, including reminder calls, letters, and emails.

- **Third-Party Collections:** As a last resort, consider using a reputable third-party collection agency for accounts that remain unpaid despite multiple attempts to collect.

7. Use of Technology

- **Automated Reminders:** Utilize automated systems for sending reminders to patients about upcoming payments or overdue balances.

- **Online Payment Portals:** Offer online payment options through patient portals, making it easier for patients to settle their bills promptly.

8. Staff Training and Patient Education

- **Staff Training:** Ensure your billing staff are well-trained in effective A/R management practices, including patient communication and negotiation of payment plans.

- **Patient Education:** Educate patients about their billing statements and payment responsibilities to reduce confusion and improve the likelihood of timely payments.

Conclusion

Effective management of accounts receivable is essential for sustaining the financial viability of healthcare practices. By implementing accurate billing practices, maintaining open lines of communication with patients, and utilizing technology for efficiency, practices can improve their A/R management, enhancing cash flow and minimizing financial risks. Regular monitoring and staff training are also vital components of a successful A/R strategy.

22.3 Financial Reporting and Analysis

Financial reporting and analysis are critical components of financial management in healthcare, providing insights into the financial health of a practice and guiding strategic decision-making. Effective financial reporting involves compiling accurate financial data into reports that are understandable and useful for stakeholders. Financial analysis then interprets these reports to evaluate financial performance and identify opportunities for improvement. Here's how to approach financial reporting and analysis in a healthcare setting.

Key Financial Reports

- **Income Statement (Profit and Loss Statement):** This report summarizes revenues, expenses, and profits over a specific period, providing insight into the practice's profitability.

- **Balance Sheet:** Offers a snapshot of the practice's financial condition at a specific point in time, detailing assets, liabilities, and equity.

- **Cash Flow Statement:** Tracks the inflow and outflow of cash, highlighting how well the practice manages its cash resources to meet its obligations.

- **Accounts Receivable Aging Report:** Shows the status of unpaid patient accounts based on the length of time the invoice has been outstanding, helping to identify potential collection issues.

Financial Analysis Techniques

- **Trend Analysis:** Involves comparing financial data over multiple periods to identify patterns, trends, and anomalies. This can help in forecasting future financial performance.

- **Ratio Analysis:** Utilizes key financial ratios, such as profit margin, return on assets, and current ratio, to assess the financial health and operational efficiency of the practice.

- **Benchmarking:** Compares the practice's financial metrics against industry standards or peers to gauge performance and identify areas for improvement.

Implementing Financial Reporting and Analysis

1. **Regular Reporting Schedule:** Establish a consistent schedule for generating and reviewing financial reports, typically monthly or quarterly, to keep stakeholders informed.

2. **Use of Financial Software:** Leverage financial management software to automate the generation of financial reports and facilitate in-depth analysis with built-in analytics tools.

3. **Training and Development:** Ensure that staff responsible for financial reporting and analysis are well-trained in accounting principles, financial management, and the use of relevant software.

4. **Stakeholder Communication:** Present financial reports and analysis findings to stakeholders in a clear, concise manner, including visual aids like charts and graphs to illustrate key points.

5. **Actionable Insights:** Translate analysis findings into actionable insights and recommendations for improving financial performance, such as cost reduction strategies, revenue enhancement opportunities, and investment considerations.

Strategic Decision-Making

- **Budgeting and Forecasting:** Use financial analysis to inform budgeting decisions and financial forecasting, anticipating future revenues, expenses, and cash flow needs.

- **Investment Decisions:** Evaluate the financial viability of potential investments, such as new technology, expansion, or hiring, based on their expected impact on the practice's financial performance.

- **Risk Management:** Identify financial risks through analysis and develop strategies to mitigate these risks, protecting the practice's financial stability.

Conclusion

Financial reporting and analysis are indispensable for the effective financial management of healthcare practices. They provide the foundation for understanding financial performance, making informed decisions, and strategizing for future growth and stability. By prioritizing accurate financial reporting and insightful analysis, healthcare providers can navigate financial challenges, capitalize on opportunities, and ensure the long-term success of their practice.

22.4 Exercise: 10 MCQs with Answers at the End

Test your knowledge on financial policy and management in healthcare, including developing a financial policy, managing accounts receivable, and financial reporting and analysis. This exercise is designed to reinforce key concepts and practices for effective financial management in a healthcare setting.

Questions:

1. What is the primary purpose of a healthcare practice's financial policy?

   A) To complicate billing processes

   B) To set clear expectations for payments and billing

C) To increase patient complaints

D) To reduce the practice's profitability

2. Accurate billing and coding primarily help to:

A) Increase claim denials

B) Reduce payment turnaround time

C) Enhance compliance and reduce errors

D) Decrease staff efficiency

3. A key component of managing accounts receivable (A/R) is:

A) Ignoring overdue accounts

B) Delaying claim submission

C) Monitoring A/R aging reports

D) Avoiding patient communication

4. Effective financial reporting in healthcare is important for:

A) Only satisfying regulatory requirements

B) Guiding strategic decision-making

C) Decreasing transparency with stakeholders

D) Complicating financial management

5. Which report provides a snapshot of a practice's financial condition at a specific point in time?

A) Income statement

B) Balance sheet

C) Cash flow statement

D) Accounts receivable aging report

6. Financial analysis can help healthcare practices:

A) Avoid planning for the future

B) Identify trends and opportunities for improvement

C) Increase financial risks

D) Reduce operational efficiency

7. Benchmarking in financial analysis involves:

A) Only focusing on internal data

B) Comparing financial metrics against industry standards

C) Ignoring peer performance

D) Decreasing competitive advantage

8. In financial management, ratio analysis is used to:

A) Simplify reporting procedures

B) Assess the financial health and operational efficiency

C) Increase financial liabilities

D) Decrease asset management effectiveness

9. Regular reviews and updates of the financial policy ensure:

A) The policy becomes outdated

B) Compliance with changing regulations

C) Reduced clarity for patients and staff

D) Increased administrative burdens

10. Offering flexible payment options to patients is a strategy to:

A) Deter timely payments

B) Improve patient satisfaction and financial outcomes

C) Overcomplicate billing processes

D) Increase unpaid debts

Answers:

1. B) To set clear expectations for payments and billing

2. C) Enhance compliance and reduce errors

3. C) Monitoring A/R aging reports

4. B) Guiding strategic decision-making

5. B) Balance sheet

6. B) Identify trends and opportunities for improvement

7. B) Comparing financial metrics against industry standards

8. B) Assess the financial health and operational efficiency

9. B) Compliance with changing regulations

10. B) Improve patient satisfaction and financial outcomes

These questions and answers aim to highlight the importance of establishing clear financial policies, effectively managing accounts receivable, and utilizing financial reporting and analysis to guide decision-making in healthcare practices. By adopting these practices, healthcare providers can ensure efficient financial management, compliance, and improved patient satisfaction.

Chapter 23: Compliance Auditing and Risk Management

23.1 Establishing a Compliance Program

In the healthcare industry, compliance is critical to ensure that practices adhere to various laws, regulations, and standards. Establishing a comprehensive compliance program is essential for minimizing risk, protecting patient information, and maintaining the integrity of billing practices. Here's a guide to setting up an effective compliance program in a healthcare setting.

Key Components of a Compliance Program

1. **Leadership and Structure:**

   - Appoint a Compliance Officer and form a compliance committee responsible for overseeing the program.

   - Ensure that the compliance program has the full support of senior management.

2. Policies and Procedures:

- Develop clear, written policies and procedures that outline compliant practices and behaviors expected of all employees.

- Include specific guidelines for billing, documentation, patient privacy (HIPAA compliance), and interactions with third-party payers.

3. Education and Training:

- Provide regular, mandatory training for all employees on compliance issues relevant to their roles.

- Update training materials regularly to reflect changes in laws and regulations.

4. Effective Communication:

- Establish open lines of communication for employees to report suspected non-compliance or ask compliance-related questions without fear of retaliation.

- Implement a confidential reporting system or hotline.

5. Monitoring and Auditing:

- Conduct regular audits and risk assessments to identify potential areas of non-compliance and evaluate the effectiveness of the compliance program.

- Use audit findings to make necessary adjustments to policies and training.

6. Enforcement and Discipline:

- Clearly outline the consequences of failing to comply with internal policies and legal requirements.

- Apply disciplinary measures fairly and consistently across the organization.

7. Response and Prevention:

- Develop a process for investigating compliance issues and implementing corrective actions.

- Use incidents of non-compliance to improve policies and prevent future violations.

Benefits of a Compliance Program

- **Risk Reduction:** Minimizes the risk of legal penalties, fines, and reputational damage associated with non-compliance.

- **Operational Efficiency:** Promotes efficient and ethical business practices that can improve operational efficiency and patient care.

- **Financial Integrity:** Ensures accurate billing and coding practices, reducing the likelihood of fraud and abuse.

- **Employee Confidence:** Builds confidence among employees that they are working in an ethical and legally compliant environment.

Steps to Establish a Compliance Program

1. **Assessment:** Start with an assessment of current practices to identify areas of risk and non-compliance.

2. **Development:** Based on the assessment, develop tailored policies and procedures to address identified risks.

3. **Implementation:** Roll out the compliance program across the organization, ensuring all staff are aware and trained.

4. **Monitoring:** Regularly monitor compliance through audits and reports, adjusting the program as necessary.

5. **Feedback Loop:** Create a feedback loop to continuously improve the compliance program based on employee input and audit outcomes.

Conclusion

Establishing a comprehensive compliance program is a proactive step towards safeguarding a healthcare practice against legal and financial risks. By fostering a culture of compliance, healthcare providers can ensure they meet regulatory requirements, protect patient information, and uphold the highest standards of ethical conduct.

23.2 Conducting Risk Assessments

Risk assessments are a critical component of a healthcare compliance program, enabling organizations to identify, analyze, and manage potential risks to their operations and compliance with laws and regulations. A well-executed risk assessment can help prevent compliance issues, financial losses, and damage to reputation. Here's how to conduct effective risk assessments in a healthcare setting.

Identify Potential Risks

1. **Billing and Coding Practices:** Evaluate the accuracy and compliance of billing and coding procedures to prevent fraud and abuse.

2. **Privacy and Security:** Assess the protection of patient health information (PHI) to ensure compliance with HIPAA and other privacy laws.

3. **Regulatory Compliance:** Identify areas where the healthcare practice may be at risk of non-compliance with healthcare laws, regulations, and standards.

4. **Operational Risks:** Examine operational processes that could lead to inefficiencies, errors, or patient safety issues.

Risk Assessment Process

1. **Establish the Scope:** Define the areas of the organization to be assessed and the objectives of the risk assessment.

2. **Gather Information:** Collect data on current practices, policies, and procedures. This may involve reviewing documentation, interviewing staff, and analyzing previous audit findings.

3. **Identify and Analyze Risks:** Identify potential risks and analyze their likelihood and potential impact on the organization. Consider factors such as the severity of consequences, the vulnerability of systems, and the effectiveness of existing controls.

4. **Prioritize Risks:** Rank identified risks based on their significance and urgency. This prioritization helps focus resources on managing the most critical risks first.

5. **Develop Mitigation Strategies:** For each identified risk, develop strategies to mitigate, transfer, avoid, or accept the risk. This may involve revising policies, implementing new controls, or providing additional training.

6. **Implement Mitigation Measures:** Put the chosen risk mitigation strategies into action. This may require allocating resources, changing processes, or updating technologies.

7. **Monitor and Review:** Regularly monitor the effectiveness of implemented measures and review the risk assessment process to identify any new risks or changes in existing risks.

Tools and Techniques

- **Risk Matrix:** Use a risk matrix to visually map the likelihood and impact of identified risks, aiding in their prioritization.

- **SWOT Analysis (Strengths, Weaknesses, Opportunities, Threats):** Utilize SWOT analysis to assess internal and external factors that could impact risk levels.

- **Checklists and Questionnaires:** Employ checklists and questionnaires to systematically identify and evaluate risks across different areas of the organization.

Documenting the Risk Assessment

- **Risk Assessment Report:** Prepare a comprehensive report detailing identified risks, analysis findings, prioritization, and recommended mitigation strategies. This report serves as a record of the assessment process and supports decision-making.

- **Action Plan:** Develop an action plan outlining the steps to be taken to address identified risks, responsible individuals, timelines, and monitoring mechanisms.

Conclusion

Conducting risk assessments is an essential practice for healthcare organizations to proactively identify and manage potential risks to their operations and compliance efforts. Through systematic identification, analysis, and mitigation of risks, healthcare providers can safeguard against compliance violations, protect patient information, and ensure the integrity of their billing practices. Regularly reviewing and updating the risk assessment process ensures that the organization can adapt to new challenges and maintain a strong compliance posture.

23.3 Implementing Corrective Actions

Implementing corrective actions is a critical step in the compliance and risk management process for healthcare organizations. Once risks have been identified and assessed, and non-compliance issues have been detected, it's essential to take systematic steps to rectify these issues and prevent their recurrence. This ensures the organization's operations align with legal and regulatory standards and protects against potential financial, legal, and reputational damage. Here's how to effectively implement corrective actions in a healthcare setting.

Identify the Root Cause

- **Thorough Investigation:** Conduct a thorough investigation of the identified compliance issue or risk to understand the underlying causes. This may involve reviewing processes, interviewing staff, and analyzing data.

- **Root Cause Analysis (RCA):** Use RCA techniques, such as the "Five Whys" method, to drill down to the fundamental cause of the problem, rather than just addressing its symptoms.

Develop a Corrective Action Plan

- **Define Specific Actions:** Based on the root cause analysis, define specific actions that need to be taken to correct the issue. These actions could range from process changes, staff retraining, policy updates, or technology improvements.

- **Assign Responsibility:** Clearly assign responsibility for each corrective action to specific individuals or teams, ensuring accountability.

- **Set Timelines:** Establish realistic timelines for implementing the corrective actions, with clear milestones and deadlines.

Implement the Actions

- **Resource Allocation:** Ensure that adequate resources (time, budget, personnel) are allocated for the implementation of corrective actions.

- **Communication:** Communicate the corrective action plan to all relevant staff, explaining the reasons for the changes and how they will be carried out.

- **Training:** If the corrective actions involve new procedures or policies, provide comprehensive training to ensure all staff understand and can comply with the changes.

Monitor and Evaluate

- **Ongoing Monitoring:** Regularly monitor the implementation of corrective actions to ensure they are being carried out as planned. Use checklists, audits, or tracking software to keep tabs on progress.

- **Evaluate Effectiveness:** After the corrective actions have been fully implemented, evaluate their effectiveness in addressing the original issue. This may involve reviewing process metrics, conducting follow-up audits, or gathering staff feedback.

- **Adjustments:** If the initial corrective actions do not fully resolve the issue or lead to unintended consequences, be prepared to make adjustments or implement additional measures.

Documentation

- **Document the Process:** Document the entire process of identifying the issue, conducting the root cause analysis, developing and implementing the corrective action plan, and evaluating its effectiveness. This documentation is crucial for accountability, future reference, and demonstrating compliance efforts to regulatory bodies.

Preventive Measures

- **Review and Update Policies:** Use the insights gained from implementing corrective actions to review and update related policies and procedures, strengthening preventive measures against future issues.

- **Continuous Improvement:** Incorporate lessons learned into the organization's continuous improvement processes, enhancing the overall compliance and risk management framework.

Conclusion

Effectively implementing corrective actions is essential for addressing compliance issues and managing risks in healthcare organizations. By identifying root causes, developing and executing a detailed corrective action plan, and monitoring its effectiveness, healthcare providers can ensure compliance, improve operational processes, and maintain high standards of care and service. This proactive approach not only addresses immediate issues but also contributes to the long-term success and sustainability of the organization.

23.4 Exercise: 10 MCQs with Answers at the End

Test your understanding of compliance auditing and risk management in healthcare, including establishing a compliance program, conducting risk assessments, and implementing corrective actions. This exercise aims to reinforce the principles and practices essential for maintaining compliance and managing risks effectively.

Questions:

1. What is the primary goal of a healthcare compliance program?

   A) To increase revenue

   B) To ensure adherence to laws and regulations

   C) To complicate operational processes

   D) To reduce staff efficiency

2. Root Cause Analysis (RCA) is used to:

   A) Identify the fundamental cause of a problem

   B) Increase the complexity of issues

   C) Assign blame to team members

   D) Ignore compliance issues

3. A key component of effective risk assessments is:

   A) Only focusing on financial risks

   B) Ignoring potential compliance issues

   C) Identifying and analyzing potential risks

   D) Conducting assessments annually

4. Corrective actions in a healthcare setting are implemented to:

A) Address and rectify identified issues

B) Overlook detected problems

C) Simplify risk management processes

D) Increase the risk of non-compliance

5. The responsibility for overseeing a compliance program typically falls to:

A) The newest staff member

B) The Compliance Officer

C) All employees equally, without a designated leader

D) External regulatory agencies

6. Effective communication in a compliance program involves:

A) Limiting information to top management

B) Establishing open lines of communication for reporting issues

C) Discouraging questions about compliance

D) Keeping compliance policies confidential

7. Monitoring and auditing within a compliance program are important for:

A) Reducing transparency and accountability

B) Identifying areas of non-compliance and evaluating the effectiveness of controls

C) Ignoring operational inefficiencies

D) Decreasing organizational awareness of compliance standards

8. When developing a corrective action plan, it's important to:

A) Avoid defining specific actions

B) Assign responsibility and set timelines

C) Delay the implementation as long as possible

D) Implement actions without monitoring their effectiveness

9. The implementation of corrective actions should include:

A) Decreasing communication with affected staff

B) Allocation of necessary resources and comprehensive training

C) Ignoring feedback from the implementation process

D) Assuming one-time actions are sufficient for long-term compliance

10. Continuous improvement in compliance and risk management involves:

  A) Repeating the same actions regardless of their effectiveness

  B) Regularly reviewing and updating policies and procedures based on lessons learned

  C) Avoiding new risk assessment strategies

  D) Maintaining static compliance and risk management programs

Answers:

1. B) To ensure adherence to laws and regulations

2. A) Identify the fundamental cause of a problem

3. C) Identifying and analyzing potential risks

4. A) Address and rectify identified issues

5. B) The Compliance Officer

6. B) Establishing open lines of communication for reporting issues

7. B) Identifying areas of non-compliance and evaluating the effectiveness of controls

8. B) Assign responsibility and set timelines

9. B) Allocation of necessary resources and comprehensive training

10. B) Regularly reviewing and updating policies and procedures based on lessons learned

These questions and answers highlight the critical components of establishing and maintaining a comprehensive compliance and risk management framework in healthcare. Through ongoing efforts in education, analysis, and corrective action, healthcare organizations can uphold high standards of compliance and minimize risks.

Chapter 24: Global Perspectives in Medical Billing

24.1 International Billing Practices

The landscape of medical billing varies significantly around the globe, influenced by differing healthcare systems, regulations, and payer models. Understanding these international billing practices offers valuable insights into the complexities of global healthcare administration and highlights the diversity in how medical services are billed and paid for across countries. Here's an overview of some key international billing practices.

United States

- **Third-Party Payers:** The U.S. healthcare system relies heavily on third-party payers, including private insurance companies, Medicare, and Medicaid. Billing involves detailed coding (ICD, CPT, HCPCS) and strict compliance with payer-specific guidelines.

- **Complexity and Variability:** The U.S. is known for its complex billing regulations, with significant variability in coverage and payment processes across different insurers.

United Kingdom

- **National Health Service (NHS):** The UK's NHS provides healthcare that is primarily funded through taxation. Medical billing practices within the NHS involve internal budgeting and funding allocations rather than billing individual patients.

- **Private Healthcare:** In the UK's private healthcare sector, billing practices more closely resemble those in the U.S., with patients directly billed for services or through private health insurance.

Canada

- **Public Healthcare System:** Canada's healthcare system is publicly funded, with provinces and territories managing their own healthcare insurance plans. Healthcare providers bill the provincial health plans directly, and patients rarely receive bills for covered services.

- **Private Insurance:** For services not covered by public health insurance, such as certain dental and vision care, private insurance or direct patient billing is used.

Germany

- **Statutory Health Insurance (SHI):** A significant portion of the German population is covered by SHI, which is funded by employer and employee contributions. Healthcare providers bill SHI schemes directly for patient services.

- **Private Health Insurance (PHI):** For those with PHI, billing can be more complex, with patients often paying upfront and seeking reimbursement from their insurer.

Japan

- **Universal Healthcare:** Japan offers universal healthcare coverage, with the government regulating prices for medical services. Patients typically pay a percentage of the cost directly to the provider, who then bills the government insurance program for the remainder.

Australia

- **Medicare:** Australia's public healthcare system, Medicare, covers many medical services and prescriptions. Providers bill Medicare directly for patient services, and patients may be responsible for a co-payment.

- **Private Insurance:** Private health insurance is also available, covering services not fully funded by Medicare, such as dental and optical services.

Emerging Trends in Global Medical Billing

- **Digitalization:** Across the globe, there is a trend toward the digitalization of medical billing processes, including the use of electronic health records (EHRs) and electronic billing systems to improve efficiency and reduce errors.

- **International Standards:** There is a growing interest in adopting international coding and billing standards to streamline the billing process, especially for multinational healthcare providers and insurers.

Conclusion

International billing practices reflect the diversity of global healthcare systems, from predominantly public-funded models offering universal coverage to systems relying heavily on private insurance. Understanding these differences is crucial for healthcare professionals working in an increasingly globalized world, as it impacts patient care, billing processes, and regulatory compliance. As the world moves toward more integrated healthcare solutions, adapting to and learning from these international practices becomes more important.

24.2 Adapting to Different Healthcare Systems

Navigating the complexities of different healthcare systems around the world requires a deep understanding of each system's unique features, funding mechanisms, and billing practices. Healthcare providers, insurers, and billing professionals must adapt their operations and services to comply with local regulations and meet the needs of patients in various regions. Here are strategies for adapting to different healthcare systems globally.

Understanding Local Healthcare Regulations

- **Research and Education:** Begin with thorough research and education on the local healthcare regulations, including coverage policies, billing procedures, and compliance requirements. This knowledge is crucial for ensuring accurate billing and avoiding legal issues.

- **Local Expertise:** Engage with local healthcare consultants or legal advisors who have in-depth knowledge of the country's healthcare laws and billing practices. They can provide valuable insights and guidance on navigating the system effectively.

Customizing Billing Processes

- **Flexible Billing Systems:** Implement billing systems that can be customized to accommodate the billing codes, formats, and submission requirements of different healthcare systems. This may involve investing in software that supports multiple languages and currencies.

- **Training Staff:** Ensure that billing staff are adequately trained on the specific billing procedures and documentation requirements of the healthcare system they are working within. Regular training updates are essential as regulations and practices evolve.

Patient Communication and Education

- **Clear Communication:** Provide clear, understandable information to patients about their rights, coverage details, and any out-of-pocket costs they may incur. This is particularly important in systems with a mix of public and private healthcare services.

- **Multilingual Support:** Offer patient communication materials and support services in multiple languages to accommodate the diverse patient population that may be accessing healthcare services in a global context.

Leveraging Technology for Efficiency

- **Electronic Health Records (EHRs):** Use EHRs to streamline patient information management and ensure that billing information is accurate and up-to-date. EHRs can also facilitate easier compliance with local data protection regulations.

- **Digital Billing and Payment Platforms:** Implement digital billing and payment solutions that allow for efficient processing of claims and payments, including the ability to handle transactions in different currencies and comply with local financial regulations.

Collaborating with Insurance Providers

- **Understanding Insurance Coverage:** Work closely with both local and international insurance providers to understand coverage policies and ensure that billing practices align with insurer requirements.

- **Direct Billing Agreements:** Establish direct billing agreements with insurers when possible, to simplify the payment process for patients and ensure timely reimbursement for services.

Fostering Cultural Competence

- **Cultural Sensitivity:** Develop cultural competence among healthcare and billing staff to ensure that services are provided in a manner that is respectful of the cultural and social norms of the patient population.

- **Customized Patient Services:** Adapt patient services and communication strategies to reflect cultural considerations, enhancing patient satisfaction and compliance with treatment and billing procedures.

Conclusion

Adapting to different healthcare systems requires a multifaceted approach that encompasses understanding local regulations, customizing billing processes, leveraging technology, and fostering cultural competence. By implementing these strategies, healthcare providers and billing professionals can effectively navigate the complexities of global healthcare, ensuring compliance, optimizing operational efficiency, and delivering high-quality patient care across different regions.

24.3 Cross-Cultural Communication Skills

Effective cross-cultural communication is essential in the global healthcare environment, where providers often interact with patients and colleagues from diverse cultural backgrounds. Misunderstandings arising from cultural differences can lead to reduced patient satisfaction, non-compliance with treatment plans, and challenges in the billing process. Enhancing cross-cultural communication skills is vital for healthcare professionals to provide inclusive care and navigate international billing practices successfully.

Understanding Cultural Differences

- **Research and Awareness:** Gain an understanding of the cultural norms, values, and communication styles of the populations you serve. Awareness of cultural differences is the first step toward effective communication.

- **Cultural Sensitivity Training:** Healthcare organizations should provide cultural sensitivity training for their staff, focusing on the nuances of verbal and non-verbal communication across cultures.

Effective Verbal Communication

- **Clear and Simple Language:** Use clear, simple language when discussing medical care and billing information. Avoid medical jargon and slang that may not be easily understood.

- **Active Listening:** Practice active listening to ensure you fully understand the patient's concerns and questions. This involves paying close attention, asking clarifying questions, and reflecting back what you have heard.

Non-Verbal Communication

- **Understanding Non-Verbal Cues:** Be aware of non-verbal communication differences, such as eye contact, facial expressions, and gestures, which can vary significantly across cultures.

- **Adapting Your Style:** Adapt your non-verbal communication style to be more in line with the patient's cultural norms, showing respect and facilitating a more comfortable interaction.

Language Assistance

- **Translation Services:** Provide access to professional translation services for patients who are not fluent in the primary language used by the healthcare provider. This can include in-person interpreters, telephone translation services, or translated materials.

- **Multilingual Staff:** Employing multilingual staff can greatly enhance communication with patients from diverse backgrounds, making them feel more understood and supported.

Building Trust and Rapport

- **Personal Connection:** Make an effort to build a personal connection with patients by showing interest in their cultural background and personal experiences. This can help build trust and improve patient engagement.

- **Patient-Centered Care:** Practice patient-centered care by respecting patients' cultural beliefs and preferences, involving them in decision-making processes, and accommodating their cultural needs whenever possible.

Navigating International Billing and Insurance

- **Cultural Considerations in Billing:** Understand cultural attitudes towards billing and insurance, including preferences for discussing financial matters and expectations around payment and insurance coverage.

- **Transparent Communication:** Clearly communicate billing policies, insurance coverage, and payment expectations, taking into account any cultural nuances that may impact the conversation.

Feedback and Continuous Learning

- **Seek Feedback:** Regularly seek feedback from patients and colleagues about your communication efforts. Use this feedback to continually improve your cross-cultural communication skills.

- **Ongoing Education:** Engage in ongoing education and training on cultural competence and cross-cultural communication to stay informed about best practices and emerging issues.

Conclusion

Developing strong cross-cultural communication skills is essential for healthcare professionals working in a global context. By understanding and respecting cultural differences, employing clear and sensitive communication strategies, and providing language assistance, healthcare providers can improve patient care, enhance patient satisfaction, and navigate the complexities of international billing practices more effectively.

24.4 Exercise: 10 MCQs with Answers at the End

Test your knowledge on global perspectives in medical billing, including international billing practices, adapting to different healthcare systems, and cross-cultural communication skills. This exercise is designed to reinforce important concepts for navigating the complexities of medical billing in a global context.

Questions:

1. In the U.S., medical billing heavily relies on:

   A) Direct government funding

   B) Third-party payers

   C) Uniform billing practices across all states

   D) Paper-based billing systems

2. The NHS in the UK primarily funds healthcare through:

   A) Out-of-pocket payments by patients

   B) Private insurance companies

C) Taxation

D) Direct billing to patients for all services

3. In Canada, healthcare providers bill:

A) Patients directly for most services

B) Provincial health plans

C) Only private insurance companies

D) International health organizations

4. Effective cross-cultural communication in healthcare involves:

A) Using medical jargon to ensure accuracy

B) Active listening and adapting communication styles

C) Avoiding discussions about cultural differences

D) Assuming all patients understand the local language perfectly

5. Cultural sensitivity training for healthcare staff focuses on:

A) The preferences of the healthcare provider

B) Understanding and respecting cultural differences

C) Promoting a single cultural standard

D) Reducing the variety of languages spoken by staff

6. The main goal of a healthcare compliance program is to:

A) Complicate billing processes

B) Ensure adherence to laws and regulations

C) Reduce staff training requirements

D) Increase operational costs

7. Root Cause Analysis (RCA) in healthcare is used to:

A) Assign blame for billing errors

B) Identify the underlying causes of issues

C) Justify non-compliance

D) Simplify legal responsibilities

8. When adapting billing processes to different healthcare systems, it is important to:

A) Apply the same procedures in every country

B) Customize billing systems to meet local requirements

C) Ignore local regulations and standards

D) Focus solely on the American healthcare model

9. Providing translation services in healthcare settings helps to:

A) Increase the complexity of medical consultations

B) Improve understanding and compliance among patients

C) Discourage learning of the local language

D) Limit the scope of services offered

10. Direct billing agreements with insurers are important for:

A) Complicating the payment process

B) Simplifying the payment process for patients

C) Increasing unpaid medical bills

D) Decreasing healthcare accessibility

Answers:

1. B) Third-party payers

2. C) Taxation

3. B) Provincial health plans

4. B) Active listening and adapting communication styles

5. B) Understanding and respecting cultural differences

6. B) Ensure adherence to laws and regulations

7. B) Identify the underlying causes of issues

8. B) Customize billing systems to meet local requirements

9. B) Improve understanding and compliance among patients

10. B) Simplifying the payment process for patients

These questions and answers aim to enhance your understanding of the diverse practices and challenges involved in medical billing across different countries, as well as the importance of effective communication and cultural sensitivity in providing healthcare services globally.

Chapter 25: The Future of Medical Billing

25.1 Trends and Predictions

The future of medical billing is being shaped by technological advancements, regulatory changes, and evolving healthcare delivery models. As the industry moves forward, several key trends and predictions are expected to redefine how billing processes are managed, enhancing efficiency, accuracy, and patient satisfaction. Here's an overview of the trends that are likely to influence the future of medical billing.

Increased Automation and AI Integration

- **Automated Billing Processes:** The use of AI and machine learning algorithms will become more prevalent in automating routine billing tasks, such as coding, claim submission, and follow-up on unpaid claims, reducing human error and increasing efficiency.

- **Predictive Analytics:** AI-driven predictive analytics will be increasingly used to forecast billing issues, such as potential claim denials, enabling preemptive corrective actions to improve the claims acceptance rate.

Blockchain for Enhanced Security and Transparency

- **Secure Transactions:** Blockchain technology is predicted to play a significant role in securing financial transactions and patient data within the billing process, offering a decentralized and tamper-proof ledger system.

- **Smart Contracts:** The use of blockchain-based smart contracts can automate billing agreements and claims processing between healthcare providers, payers, and patients, streamlining workflows and reducing administrative overhead.

Telehealth and Remote Services Billing

- **Expanded Coverage:** As telehealth services continue to grow, billing codes and insurance policies will evolve to provide comprehensive coverage for remote healthcare services, standardizing telehealth billing practices.

- **Remote Patient Monitoring (RPM):** Billing for RPM services will become more common, with specific codes and reimbursement models developed to support this mode of patient care.

Interoperability and Data Integration

- **Seamless Data Exchange:** Enhanced interoperability among EHR systems, billing software, and payer systems will facilitate seamless data exchange, improving billing accuracy and reducing claim denials.

- **Consolidated Platforms:** The development of consolidated platforms that integrate clinical, administrative, and financial data will provide a unified view of patient information, streamlining the billing process.

Patient-Centric Billing

- **Transparent Pricing:** There will be a greater emphasis on price transparency, with healthcare providers offering clear and upfront cost estimates to patients before services are rendered.

- **Digital Payment Options:** The adoption of digital and mobile payment options will increase, making it easier for patients to understand, manage, and pay their healthcare bills.

Regulatory Compliance and Quality Reporting

- **Value-Based Care:** The shift towards value-based care models will continue, requiring billing processes to adapt to new reimbursement structures that focus on patient outcomes and cost efficiency.

- **Quality Reporting:** Compliance with quality reporting requirements will become more integrated into the billing process, linking reimbursement more closely with the quality of care provided.

Globalization of Healthcare Services

- **International Billing Standards:** As healthcare becomes more globalized, there may be a push towards developing international billing standards to simplify billing for cross-border healthcare services.

- **Cultural Competence:** Billing practices will need to become more culturally competent, accommodating the needs of a diverse global patient population.

Conclusion

The future of medical billing is poised for significant transformation, driven by technological innovations, regulatory changes, and shifts in patient expectations. By staying abreast of these trends and adapting to the evolving landscape, healthcare providers and billing professionals can ensure they are well-positioned to meet the challenges and opportunities that lie ahead, ultimately improving the efficiency and effectiveness of medical billing processes.

25.2 Preparing for Changes in Healthcare

As the healthcare industry continues to evolve, driven by technological advancements, regulatory changes, and shifting patient expectations, healthcare organizations and professionals must be prepared to adapt. Preparing for these changes is crucial for maintaining operational efficiency, ensuring compliance, and providing high-quality patient care. Here's how healthcare entities can brace themselves for the ongoing and future shifts in the healthcare landscape.

Stay Informed on Industry Trends

- **Continuous Learning:** Commit to ongoing education and training to stay abreast of the latest developments in healthcare technology, billing practices, and regulatory requirements.

- **Industry Engagement:** Participate in healthcare industry groups, associations, and forums to exchange knowledge and experiences with peers.

Invest in Technology

- **Adopt Advanced Solutions:** Invest in advanced healthcare IT solutions, including EHR systems, billing software, and telehealth platforms that offer scalability and flexibility to adapt to new healthcare delivery models.

- **Embrace Automation:** Leverage automation and AI technologies to streamline administrative tasks, reduce errors, and improve efficiency in billing and patient care processes.

Enhance Data Security and Compliance

- **Strengthen Data Protection:** Implement robust cybersecurity measures to protect patient data and comply with privacy regulations such as HIPAA in the U.S. or GDPR in Europe.

- **Regular Compliance Audits:** Conduct regular compliance audits and risk assessments to identify areas of vulnerability and ensure adherence to current healthcare laws and standards.

Cultivate a Flexible Organizational Culture

- **Promote Adaptability:** Foster a culture of flexibility and adaptability among staff, encouraging innovation and open-mindedness to change.

- **Support Staff Training:** Provide comprehensive training and professional development opportunities to equip staff with the skills needed to navigate changes in healthcare practices and technologies.

Focus on Patient-Centric Care

- **Improve Patient Engagement:** Implement strategies to enhance patient engagement and satisfaction, such as improving communication, offering patient portals, and providing transparent billing practices.

- **Adapt to Patient Needs:** Be prepared to adjust operational practices to meet changing patient expectations, such as the demand for more remote care options and digital health services.

Develop Strategic Partnerships

- **Collaborate with Technology Providers:** Form strategic partnerships with technology providers and other healthcare organizations to leverage shared resources, knowledge, and innovations.

- **Engage with Payers:** Work closely with insurance companies and payers to understand changes in reimbursement models and ensure alignment with billing practices.

Plan for Financial Sustainability

- **Diversify Revenue Streams:** Explore new revenue opportunities, such as offering additional healthcare services or adopting alternative payment models like value-based care.

- **Optimize Resource Allocation:** Continually assess and optimize the allocation of resources to ensure financial sustainability amidst changing healthcare economics.

Conclusion

Preparing for changes in healthcare requires a proactive and strategic approach, focusing on education, technology adoption, compliance, organizational flexibility, patient-centric care, strategic partnerships, and financial planning. By embracing these strategies, healthcare organizations can navigate the complexities of the evolving healthcare landscape, ensuring they remain resilient, compliant, and focused on delivering exceptional patient care.

25.3 Innovations in Medical Billing

The medical billing landscape is undergoing significant transformation, driven by technological advancements and the need for more efficient, transparent, and patient-centered processes. Innovations in medical billing are not only streamlining administrative tasks but also enhancing the accuracy of billing, improving patient satisfaction, and enabling healthcare providers to focus more on patient care. Here's a look at some of the key innovations shaping the future of medical billing.

Automated Billing Systems

- **AI and Machine Learning:** AI algorithms and machine learning are increasingly being used to automate complex billing tasks, such as coding and claims processing. These technologies can analyze vast amounts of data to identify patterns, predict denials, and suggest corrective actions, thereby reducing errors and improving claim acceptance rates.

Blockchain Technology

- **Secure Data Exchange:** Blockchain offers a secure and transparent way to store and exchange data, including patient records and billing information. Its application in medical billing can reduce fraud, enhance data security, and streamline the reconciliation and settlement processes between payers and providers.

- **Smart Contracts:** Blockchain-based smart contracts can automatically execute agreements based on predefined rules, such as verifying insurance eligibility or processing claims, reducing manual intervention and speeding up transactions.

Electronic Health Records (EHR) Integration

- **Seamless Workflow:** Integrating billing systems with EHRs enables seamless data flow, reducing the need for duplicate data entry and minimizing errors. This integration ensures that billing information is accurate and up-to-date, reflecting the patient's latest medical records.

- **Real-Time Eligibility Checks:** Advanced EHR systems offer real-time insurance eligibility checks and pre-authorization features, helping providers understand coverage details and reduce the incidence of claim rejections.

Telehealth Billing Solutions

- **Dedicated Telehealth Codes:** As telehealth becomes a mainstay in healthcare delivery, billing solutions are evolving to include dedicated telehealth billing codes and reimbursement models. These solutions facilitate the accurate billing of telehealth services, ensuring providers are compensated appropriately.

- **Remote Patient Monitoring (RPM):** Billing for RPM services is becoming more streamlined, with specific codes and guidelines that recognize the value of remote care in patient management.

Patient-Centric Billing Platforms

- **Transparent Pricing Tools:** Online tools and platforms that offer transparent pricing and cost estimates empower patients to understand their financial responsibilities before receiving services, improving transparency and trust.

- **Digital Payment Options:** The adoption of digital wallets, online payment portals, and mobile payment apps simplifies the payment process for patients, offering convenience and flexibility in managing their healthcare expenses.

Analytics and Reporting Tools

- **Data-Driven Insights:** Advanced analytics and reporting tools provide healthcare organizations with insights into billing patterns, payer behavior, and revenue cycle performance. These tools help identify areas for improvement, optimize billing processes, and enhance financial decision-making.

Regulatory Compliance Software

- **Automated Compliance Checks:** Software solutions that automatically check for compliance with billing regulations and standards can help healthcare providers avoid costly penalties and ensure that billing practices adhere to legal requirements.

Conclusion

Innovations in medical billing are revolutionizing how healthcare providers manage financial transactions, comply with regulations, and engage with patients regarding their billing. By leveraging these technologies and solutions, healthcare organizations can achieve greater efficiency, accuracy, and patient satisfaction, paving the way for a more sustainable and patient-focused healthcare system.

25.4 Exercise: 10 MCQs with Answers at the End

Test your knowledge on the future of medical billing, focusing on trends, innovations, and strategies for adapting to changes in healthcare. This exercise is designed to reinforce key concepts and insights into evolving practices in medical billing.

Questions:

1. Which technology is increasingly used to automate billing tasks and improve claim accuracy?

   A) Typewriters

   B) Fax machines

   C) AI and machine learning

   D) Pagers

2. Blockchain technology in medical billing enhances:

   A) Data insecurity

   B) Transparency and data security

   C) Manual reconciliation processes

   D) Paper-based recordkeeping

3. Integration of billing systems with EHRs primarily aims to:

   A) Increase manual data entry

   B) Reduce data accuracy

   C) Streamline data flow and reduce errors

   D) Complicate the billing process

4. Dedicated telehealth billing codes are developed to:

   A) Discourage telehealth services

   B) Ensure appropriate reimbursement for telehealth services

   C) Increase billing complexity for telehealth

   D) Limit access to telehealth services

5. Patient-centric billing platforms focus on:

   A) Decreasing payment options

   B) Obscuring pricing information

   C) Enhancing transparency and providing digital payment options

   D) Promoting paper billing statements

6. Real-time insurance eligibility checks benefit healthcare providers by:

   A) Increasing claim rejections

   B) Reducing administrative efficiency

   C) Helping to prevent claim denials

   D) Eliminating the need for insurance

7. Smart contracts in blockchain technology automate:

A) Data breaches

B) Billing agreements and claims processing

C) Manual data entry

D) Compliance violations

8. Analytics and reporting tools in medical billing are used to:

A) Ignore financial data

B) Provide insights into billing patterns and revenue cycle performance

C) Reduce data-driven decision-making

D) Simplify regulatory compliance

9. The adoption of digital and mobile payment options in medical billing aims to:

A) Limit patient payment methods

B) Simplify the payment process for patients

C) Increase unpaid medical bills

D) Discourage timely payments

10. Automated compliance checks in billing software help to:

A) Increase legal penalties

B) Ensure adherence to billing regulations

C) Complicate compliance efforts

D) Reduce software functionality

Answers:

1. C) AI and machine learning

2. B) Transparency and data security

3. C) Streamline data flow and reduce errors

4. B) Ensure appropriate reimbursement for telehealth services

5. C) Enhancing transparency and providing digital payment options

6. C) Helping to prevent claim denials

7. B) Billing agreements and claims processing

8. B) Provide insights into billing patterns and revenue cycle performance

9. B) Simplify the payment process for patients

10. B) Ensure adherence to billing regulations

These questions and answers highlight the emerging trends and innovations in medical billing, emphasizing the importance of technology in enhancing efficiency, security, and patient satisfaction in healthcare financial management.

Conclusion

As we've explored the multifaceted aspects of medical billing, from foundational knowledge and best practices to global perspectives and future trends, it's clear that the field is both complex and dynamic. The evolution of medical billing is driven by technological advancements, regulatory changes, and the shifting landscape of healthcare delivery. To navigate these changes successfully, healthcare professionals and billing specialists must stay informed, adaptable, and patient-focused.

Key Takeaways:

1. **Comprehensive Knowledge:** Understanding the core principles of medical billing, including coding, insurance processes, and patient communication, is crucial for accuracy and efficiency.

2. **Adaptability:** The ability to adapt to changes in healthcare regulations, billing practices, and technology is essential for maintaining compliance and optimizing billing processes.

3. **Technological Proficiency:** Leveraging technology, such as EHR integration, AI, and blockchain, can significantly enhance the efficiency and security of billing operations.

4. **Global Awareness:** Recognizing and adapting to the diverse billing practices and healthcare systems around the world is important for professionals involved in global healthcare services.

5. **Future-Oriented:** Anticipating and preparing for future trends, including the rise of telehealth billing and patient-centric platforms, will ensure that healthcare organizations remain competitive and responsive to patient needs.

6. **Continuous Improvement:** Ongoing education, training, and professional development are vital for keeping up with the evolving field of medical billing.

By embracing these principles, healthcare providers and billing professionals can ensure that they not only meet the current demands of the healthcare industry but are also well-prepared for the challenges and opportunities that lie ahead. The future of medical billing promises greater efficiency, transparency, and patient satisfaction, driven by innovation and a commitment to excellence in healthcare financial management.

The best way to thank an author is to

write a review.